THE COMPLETE GUIDE TO

Rick Kiddle

STUDIO CYCLING

1st edition

A & C Black • London

Note

Whilst every effort has been made to ensure that the content of this book is as technically accurate and as sound as possible, neither the editors nor the publishers can accept responsibility for any injury or loss sustained as a result of the use of this material

Published by A & C Black Publishers Ltd
37 Soho Square, London W1D 3QZ
www.acblack.com

ISBN 0 7136 6462 2

A CIP catalogue record for this book is available from the British Library.

Acknowledgements
Cover photograph © Grant Pritchard
Photographs © Grant Pritchard

A & C Black uses paper produced with elemental chlorine-free pulp, harvested from managed sustainable forests.

Typeset in 10½ on 12pt Baskerville BE Regular

Printed and bound in Great Britain by Biddles Ltd, Kings Lynn

CONTENTS

Foreword   vii

Preface   viii

Introduction What is Studio Cycling?   ix

 1 Health and Fitness   1

 2 Getting Started   5

 3 Visualisation, Focus and Concentration   38

 4 Heart Zone Training for Studio Cycling   48

 5 General Training Zones within a Class Structure   59

 6 Further Assistance for Instructors   87

 7 Different Forms of Studio Cycling   113

 8 Studio Cycling at Home   123

 9 Athletes 'Spin to Win'   135

10 Overtraining   136

11 Special Populations   139

Glossary   160

References   161

Index   162

DEDICATION

This book is dedicated to my son Niall, whose name means 'champion' and 'passionate', the characteristics that make someone want to be the best they can. I don't care what sport (if any) he is good at, just as long as, if he does follow a dream – like I have all my life – he works hard, practises, and does his best – which is all anyone can ever ask.

Thanks

A massive 'thank you' goes to my friends at Heart Zones and Schwinn. I have been made to feel part of their families. From them I continue to follow a path of learning and growth.

This book wouldn't have been possible without the help from two people: Georgina Heron, who spent days and nights sifting through my ramblings on the computer; together we came out with something that made sense; and Chris Mackie, who has helped to keep me in one piece by taking the pressure off when it has been most intense. A special mention must be made of Tony, who helped with the profiles, and there are hundreds of other people who I would like to thank personally for inspiration and guidance – but not in this book, because the readers probably want to get on and start riding, just like I do when the sun is shining!

Rick Kiddle

ACKNOWLEDGMENTS

When I think about cycling and what it means to me, it has to symbolise freedom! The freedom to be an individual and express myself. There are three people I would like to acknowledge who have helped me find freedom with my cycling. When I was just fourteen years old I went youth hostelling to Norfolk and the New Forest. This was the first time I had ever left home and had no one looking after me or keeping me in line. I would like to thank my mum and dad for allowing me to go, believing in me that I would be safe and mature enough as a young teenager. They have supported me through thick and thin all my life, they still are and I have the best parents a son could ever want.

I think writing a book takes a bit of front to be honest. You are basically saying that what I have to say is good enough for everyone to hear, especially one's peers. Rod Markwell, the owner of a sports retail business (who unfortunately passed away many years ago) changed my whole perception of myself when I was 21 years old. Without realising it he allowed me to focus on what I really wanted to get out of my sport; because of him I set out a long term plan to achieve athletic goals that had previously seemed like dreams with no reality. Becoming an international Triathlete and winning the National Championships gave me the confidence in my own ability that will last me a lifetime because no one could ever take those things away from me. Just like no-one can ever take this achievement of writing a book away from me. Now it is written I can start a new chapter in my life, although it will somehow be connected to a bike!

FOREWORD

If you are new to cycling, Rick Kiddle's *The Complete Guide to Studio Cycling* is the best tool you could have to achieve success. If you are an experienced indoor cyclist, read this to hone your skills and learn the latest on training, bike fit and so much more. Kiddle, one of the world's leading authorities on studio cycling, shares more than his expertise and experiences with the reader. He shows you how to do it clearly and correctly in a motivational way for every level of rider.

For the past 25 years, Rick has been riding, racing and simultaneously teaching others the tricks of his trade. Few coaches or teachers are successful at both at the same time. Most professionals can only do one at a time – either teach or race. Kiddle is the exception. He has the ability to master both at the same time. Possibly it's an athlete's ego that prevents him or her from sharing what they are so good at with others. Or, maybe it's a sense that there are secrets that a rider should not share with others; as if there's magic in what it takes to cross the finish line in first place. But Rick proves the fallacy in this as, even today, he continues to race, run his own studio cycling business and write this, his first book, with articulacy.

When I first met Rick, I was leading a Heart Zones Training seminar in the UK and he approached me with a simple inquiry – would I share with him everything about how to train using the heart muscle as the core of a goal-oriented training system? I admire those who start a relationship by asking the hard questions. Although he had been training and racing in professional triathlons for decades, he still knew, as most of us do, that there is always more to learn. Rick knows that there is not just one way to ride or just one way to train. Quickly, Rick mastered Heart Zones and started to teach others one of the most cutting-edge ways to ride which is individualised to each person's fitness preferences.

But, more than training, Rick presents the complete information on mental focus, how to organise a studio cycling class, training at home, how to get started and advanced techniques. If you are the type that wants to get it all in one book, *The Complete Guide to Studio Cycling* is the one to start with. And, if you are like the tens of thousands of individuals who Rick has trained over these past two decades, you will know why the guy is a master – his passion is that you get great on the bike. You will quickly discover that his love for riding becomes your love for riding. He is the expert and his goal is for you to be a constantly improving rider.

In the Japanese language, improving using 'kaizen' is the standard. Kaizen means small, constant improvement. It is a way of getting better by improving 1 per cent a hundred times. In contrast, many riders try to take the giant leap of one effort that leads to a 100 per cent change. The giant leap usually falls short and leads to crashing into a chasm. But Rick shows you step-by-step how to ride the bike with more efficiency, with less effort and with more joy. He shows you how to kaizen your riding experience by giving you hundreds of ways to improve 1 per cent each time.

If you want to improve your riding 100 per cent, then get out your yellow highlighter and start reading *The Complete Guide to Studio Cycling*. I warn you in advance, you are going to be underlining pages and pages as you digest each chapter and the 'Kiddle' way of riding better.

After all, isn't that what you want as you gain riding proficiency? The best way that I know of to improve is to educate yourself, learn from the master, and spend a lot of time in the saddle burning calories, feeling the sensation of getting fitter and faster, and gaining the benefits of fitness training on a bike. And, there's more – read on and ride on.

Sally Edwards, author, professional athlete,
and founder of Heart Zones Training
Sacramento, California
January 2004
www.HeartZones.com

PREFACE

Studio cycling appeals to all ages and abilities because it is run within a controlled environment on a stationary bike specially designed *not* to measure one individual against another, whilst at the same time allowing each person within the group to develop their fitness at their own pace.

It can be sociable, fun and inexpensive. This new, fast-growing way of training can certainly ensure optimum fitness! Cycling is one of Britain's favourite pastimes and modes of transport, one adult in every three owns a bike (Mintel, 1995; www.bikebiz.co.uk) with around a third of the users commuting on their bikes. Studio cycling can help more people like this to enjoy cycling in company, instead of leaving their bikes rusting and lonely in the garage. Simple training will produce fitness, technique and confidence, and so studio cycling can change lives for everyone's benefit.

Fact: If one-third of all short journeys now made in a car were made by bike instead, rates of national heart disease would fall by between 5 and 10 per cent (*Bikes not Fumes*, CTC, 1992). This is why encouraging studio cyclists out onto the road has to be a major goal.

INTRODUCTION – WHAT IS STUDIO CYCLING?

History

Studio cycling originated with Johnny Goldberg in California in the early 1990s. The concept of getting groups of people to train together on bikes wasn't original, but in the studio it was new and different and proved highly successful, and a new phenomenon called Spinning® was born. Once a major manufacturer (Schwinn) was found who could make the special bikes it was only a matter of time and hard work by Johnny at US fitness industry trade shows. Soon over 300 clubs up and down America were running successful Spinning programmes on Schwinn. The sport was driven by the personality and enthusiasm of the originator and his style of delivery took the industry by storm. In Europe people were a

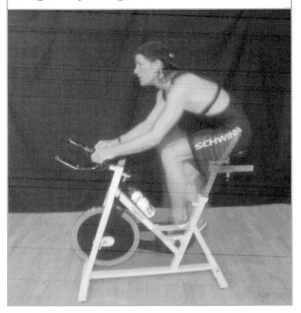

Original Spinning bike

little more sceptical and needed further proof that it wasn't to be a short-lived fad. Many clubs waited until the evidence showed the benefits of fitter people therefore aiding membership retention and mass participation. The classes, however, were only as strong as the instructors and so an education process was needed to teach the instructors how to run these special classes. The Schwinn-run programme led the way, but soon dozens of imitations sprang up with their own form of training. Imitation is the best form of flattery, so this was proof of a strong programme or concept; however, the imitators have in some ways lost track of the goals and purpose of the original concept of training, and how it should be run, because many don't come from a cycling background. The results of over 100 years of experimenting with cycling training and programmes can't be wrong: cyclists and cycling coaches know how a bike should be ridden, and the new concept of bringing road cycling indoors has opened the way for further development of an already existing structure of training. In this book we intend to build on this and give you more exciting ideas to use, develop and further your training.

The idea of cycling indoors is not new. Cyclists themselves developed training on machines called Rollers and Turbo Trainers where they could ride their own bikes within their own training programme.

These machines have been limited to competitive cyclists with goals as they can be boring and demotivating. Indeed most fitness clubs have some form of indoor bikes for cardiovascular training in or around their gym areas, although it is rare to find anyone who can manage to use one for more than ten minutes

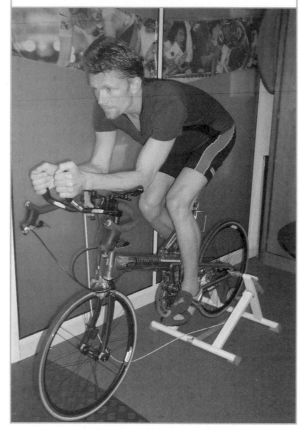

Author on turbo Airnimal bike

before they lose interest and move on to the next machine.

This book is intended to answer all your questions and take you on your own journey towards fitness and health; whether you are new to fitness or a competitive cyclist read on and enjoy – you may even become a stronger cyclist!

Readers' profile

Studio cycling is for everyone! It has grown from the fitness industry, where millions of people every day are now using the concept to reach their goals. Are you one of them?

Health benefits of cycling

Regular cyclists enjoy a fitness level equal to that of a person ten years younger (Sharp National Forum for Coronary Heart Disease Foundation).

Cycling at least 20 miles a week (approximately two studio-cycling classes; NSCR 2003) reduces the risk of heart disease to less than half that for non-cyclists who take no other exercise (Morris British Heart Foundation) (www.bikebiz.co.uk).

We believe if you are seeking to incorporate any level of cardiovascular fitness into your training then studio cycling will fit into your programme. All can benefit, from serious cyclists who can shelter indoors away from the elements such as cold, dark, rainy nights, icy roads and short daylight hours and still get exactly the same benefits as if riding on roads or trails, to anyone who would profit from measuring and monitoring themselves in a safe environment. People who are scared of riding on dangerous roads or don't have the basic balance and skill to ride a bike with two wheels can ride a bike with one! You may not move or go anywhere, but you can become extremely fit.

In the area of weight loss studio cycling has revolutionised the fitness industry. Men and women who have previously been bored with their training can now enjoy classes, see amazing results and follow a safe and structured programme, speeding the metabolic rate and burning fat like no other exercise class. The nature of studio cycling is that it brings road cycling indoors, people can go on a mental bike journey, however with the clever design of the bike it means that even the most novice unfit cyclist can ride next to the professional and the elderly can ride next to the young. Teams can enjoy training together and the coach can incorporate specific goals for whole teams and individuals in such sports as: football, rugby, hockey, cricket, basketball, swimming, golf, running, boxing, martial arts, netball, volleyball, triathlon, gymnastics, duathlon, biathlon, darts, hurling, curling . . . the list becomes endless.

The chapters of this book will help you to find ideas, concepts, techniques, profiles, and programmes that will aid you with your training. Studio cycling is simply for everyone.

Choose your programme for: Mind (focusing, concentration); Body (weight loss, fat loss, strength, endurance, power, rehabilitation); Cardiovascular heart rate training (juniors and seniors); Team sports (football, rugby, etc.); Individual sports (running, cycling, etc.)

The concept of studio cycling

Studio cycling is an individualised training programme within a group. It brings the ideas

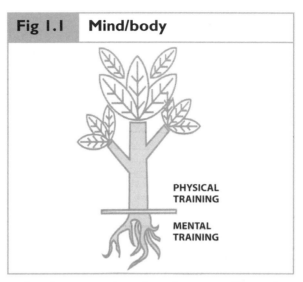

Fig 1.1 **Mind/body**

PHYSICAL TRAINING

MENTAL TRAINING

and techniques of road cycling into the studio, using stationary bikes with a fixed flywheel. Each rider trains at his or her own level by adding resistance with an uncalibrated braking mechanism. If this all sounds a little technical it will become clearer as you read on.

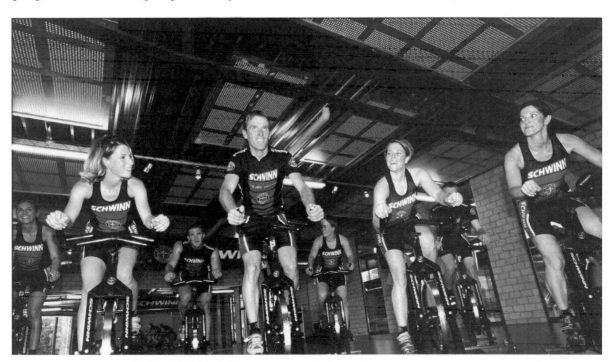

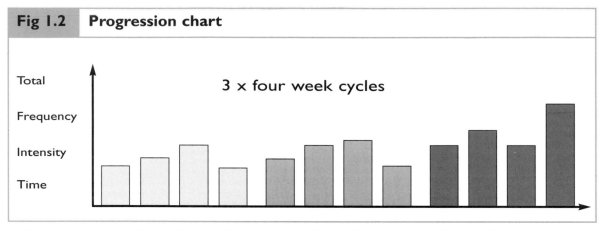

Fig 1.2 Progression chart

3 x four week cycles

Total

Frequency

Intensity

Time

Classes are run with multiples of bikes from as many as 5 to 100; as you can imagine, the more people you have the better – it allows you to get lost in the crowd, or focus on your own training, or enjoy the beauty of the motivation from others around you. However, if space is an issue five bikes could easily be placed in the corner of the gym. At fitness conventions there have been as many as 400 bikes in one venue! The classes themselves are run with an instructor or coach who leads the class through a workout to music. There are three elements to each class:

1 Fun, motivation and high energy.
2 Mental training including focusing techniques.
3 Training programme with progression.

Why choose studio cycling?

Many people choose cycling as an exercise for numerous reasons but perhaps one of the biggest advantages is that it is a non-load-bearing exercise, where the joints are put under less stress than in running, and no doubt that is one of the reasons that studio cycling has become so popular. Also you are able to control your own training session and work at your own pace within a group.

Benefits of studio cycling – both indoors and outdoors

The benefits of studio cycling need little explanation. If you are already a road cyclist or mountain biker you will certainly be aware of the negatives of riding outside: you need only think of those winter days when the light draws in by the time you leave work, it's blowing a gale and the rain is lashing down; the thought of doing a turbo training session would more than likely bore even the keenest cyclist to tears. This is when cyclists find their way to a studio cycling class. It has all the advantages: it is dry, warm and light and allows you to ride at your own pace in a group while at the same time being motivated and improving your cycling technique and strength. What started as a seasonal functional training session becomes an all-round routine scheduled into even the most competitive cyclist training programme.

Of course you don't have to be a cyclist to enjoy the benefits; you don't even have to be particularly fit – that is something that will progress if you continue to follow the training programme set by your instructor. So whether your goal is weight loss, body toning or just simply getting fitter, studio cycling will help you achieve it.

HEALTH AND FITNESS

The definition of fitness is to be in good health or condition, and therefore this is not a performance rating. How many times have you heard people say, 'I'd love to join a studio cycling class but I'm not fit enough'? The answer to that is that no one is 'not fit enough' to spin; the instructor does not force you to put the resistance onto the flywheel – it is something that you do yourself. Fitness comes later when you allow yourself to be challenged in a class. This chapter on health and fitness will aid you on the way to a healthy mind and fitter body.

If you are going to separate the performance rating of individuals then you must also create different classes for experience and capability, which is why it is necessary to have varied types of class for people to choose from. This choice must be made by the class member in the first instance; however, ultimately the instructor should place the person in a suitable class.

Nutrition

Have you ever heard the phrase, 'We are what we eat'? It is a true statement: a healthy diet will result in improvements in energy levels, muscle strength, hair, skin, nails and all-round well-being. In order to follow a healthy diet it is important to have a certain element of knowledge about the food you eat; this chapter aims to help you, not by telling you what you are to eat but by explaining why and how your diet can help you adapt to exercise.

The balance of a daily diet should be approximately: 50–60% carbohydrates; 25–30% fat; 15–20% protein. Men should consume 2500 kcal per day, and women 2000 kcal per day (the more exercise the higher the consumption).

Eating before and during exercise

Many people are nervous about what to eat before exercise or a race. However, fuelling your body is vital to performance especially prior to a long ride or race. Ideally you should eat at least 1–2 hours before exercise; your food intake should consist primarily of complex carbohydrate such as porridge, pasta or rice with some protein. It is important not to eat food that is high in fat and sugar as your body will be unable to digest it.

Why eat carbohydrate before exercise?

Carbohydrates can take on many different forms. Monosaccharide units can pair up to form diasaccharides, or join up in longer chains to form oligosaccharides or polysaccharides.

Insulin 'removes' the glucose from the blood. The glucose is transported into the muscles and into the fatty tissue. When our glycogen stores are well fuelled by a diet rich in carbohydrate, we can exert ourselves for a longer period of time.

> If we have a diet rich in carbohydrate our glycogen stores will be replenished and we will be ready to train within 12–24 hours. However if we have a diet rich in protein and fat the process will take 2–3 days.

Table 1.1	Types of carbohydrate		
	Examples	**Found in**
Monosaccharides (monoses)	Glucose Fructose Galactose	Honey Fruit Milk
Diasaccharides (dioses)	Saccharose Maltose Lactose	Sugar Malt Drink Milk
Ogliosaccharides up to 10 monosaccharide units	Maltotroise Dextrin	Toast, crisp bread etc
Polysaccharide (complex carbs.) more than ten up to several 100,000s of monosaccharide units	Vegetable starch Animal glycogen	Cereals Breads Rice

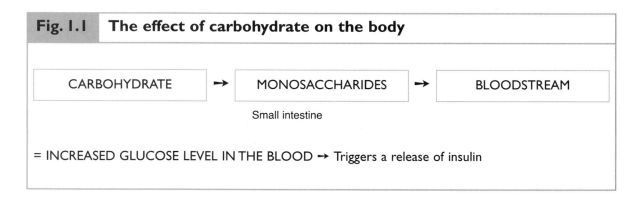

Fig. 1.1	The effect of carbohydrate on the body

CARBOHYDRATE → MONOSACCHARIDES → BLOODSTREAM

Small intestine

= INCREASED GLUCOSE LEVEL IN THE BLOOD → Triggers a release of insulin

Are any fats acceptable in our diet?

Yes, fats are just as important as carbohydrate and protein. Just as it is important that your training should be balanced, so should your diet. There are many different types of fats. The fatty acids are differentiated according to their length (short-chain, medium-chain, long-chain) and according to whether they are saturated or unsaturated.

Fat plays an important role in the body; it lubricates joints, protects internal organs and is a concentrated source of energy.

BAD FATS = Saturated fats	• Increased cholesterol level • Contained in animal fats such as meat, milk products, cheese and butter
'IN MODERATION' FATS = Monosaturated fats	• Liquid consistency • Positive effects on cholesterol levels • Contained in vegetable oils, such as olive oil and peanut oil
GOOD FATS = Polyunsaturated fats	• Liquid consistency • Positive effect on cholesterol • Vegetable oils • Fish — herring, mackerel, and salmon

What about protein?

When you think of a diet high in protein it might bring to mind pictures of bodybuilders drinking protein shakes and devouring huge steaks. As a result you might think it is better to cut back on your intake of protein rather than increase it. Actually this is not true: you could be denying your body vital nutrients since body proteins break down when you exercise or participate in any other heavy muscular activity. Twenty per cent of the body consists of protein. Emphasis is often placed on carbohydrates when it comes to health and fitness, but protein also plays a vital role in building and repairing muscles, and maintaining all types of tissue; it helps to keep brain cells functioning and the blood flowing. Even more high-quality protein is needed if you are exercising. Some of the symptoms of lack of protein are chronic fatigue, constant colds or general weakness.

Every cell in your body contains protein, formed by the body breaking down the bulk protein you eat in your food and creating compounds called amino acids.

Proteins are essential for:
• energy;
• hormones to control metabolism;
• the repair, structure and definition of muscles;
• resistance to illness;
• the repair and maintenance of tissue.

The Recommended Daily Allowance (RDA) for protein:

0.8 grams of protein per kilogram of body weight
OR
0.36 grams of protein per pound of weight.

The RDA does not represent a minimum standard but instead a level of protein that has a built-in safety factor, calculated to meet the needs of virtually all healthy people in the population. Bear in mind that hard-training athletes may need more.

Exercise initially weakens your body, depleting energy stores and damaging muscle and connective tissue. Perhaps this is the reason that nutrition and refuelling the body become so important. Recovery is a rebuilding process. It is during this period that your body is refuelled, helping to repair connective tissue and make muscles stronger. Improvements in strength and endurance are not made during exercise but during recovery. To maximise fitness goals and achieve them, your exercise intensity must be in balance with your recovery. However, the recovery process can be lengthy, resulting in frustration for athletes in training who find they have a lack of energy, inconsistent workouts, slow or no improvement and a tendency to injury. In order to aid the body in this recovery process, it needs the correct nutrients. The body recovers at the greatest rate within two hours of finish of the exercise.

Athletes and energy

Endurance strains the muscles, which decreases muscular protein. Carbohydrates are economic fuel for our muscles because they feed red blood cells and require less oxygen for combustion. Fat is the long-term fuel provider for our muscles but requires a lot of oxygen. Fats and carbohydrates supplement each other in our energy metabolism.

Diets are a short-term solution to losing fat weight. The safest and most reliable way is to change your intake of foods and lead an active life. Here are our recommendations:

- Eat low-fat food
  - Cut down on animal fats
  - Prepare low-fat foods
- Eat sufficient complex carbohydrates
  - Eat foods rich in dietary fibres, (wholegrain) cereal products etc.
- Eat fewer sweets and sugary foods
- Eat plenty of cooked vegetables, fruit and salads (low-fat dressings)
- Drink at least 1.5 litres of liquid (water) per day
  - Drink mineral water, herbal teas, juices (not concentrated)
- Lack of water has a dramatic influence on our performance, causing
  - Circulation trouble
  - Reduced transport of nutrients and oxygen
  - Muscle weakness, cramps
- Decrease in performance
- Collapse
- Never wait till you are thirsty before you drink
- Pick foods with a high density of nutrients, with
  - Little fat, and lots of vitamins, minerals and dietary fibres.

Vitamins ('vita' means 'life') are regulators of our metabolism, they act as co-factors of enzymes. Our body cannot produce them so we must take them in through the food and drink we consume. Minerals that fulfil important functions in our body, are lost in sweat.

Have your last big meal 2–3 hours before training and competition. Light snacks (bananas, dried fruit, toast, etc.) can be eaten up to 30 minutes beforehand. You can eat bananas or energy bars during exercise but try them in training before you use them in competition. Drink in small amounts, about 100–200ml of water or juices mixed with water. For exertion longer than 60 minutes ingest a maximum of 65g of carbohydrates per hour depending on intensity.

After training or competition: Drink carbohydrate-rich drinks, eat carbohydrate snacks within the first two hours of finishing. After an endurance class or marathon spin, eat up to 100g of carbohydrates, then eat high-quality protein to regenerate the strained muscles.

GETTING STARTED

Whether you are buying your own bike or simply joining a class there are a few things that may help you to have a more comfortable ride.

Buying the right bike

Purchasing a studio cycling bike is not something that you should rush into; there are a lot of manufacturers in the industry who are not so concerned with the cost or set up of their bikes.

Fig. 2.1	Studio-cycling bike

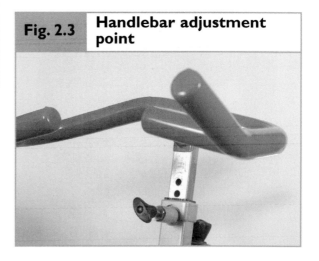

Some helpful hints on buying the right bike are:
- check for comfort, especially the touch points: saddles, handlebars, pedals (see Fig. 2.2)
- Find a bike that has maximum adjustments – just like a road bike, it should be adjustable to suit you (see Fig. 2.3).

Fig. 2.2	Touch points: saddle, handlebars and pedals

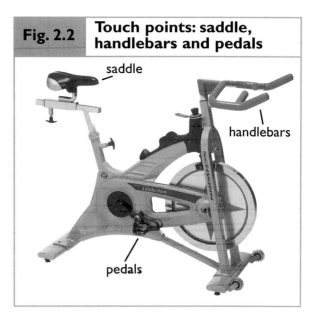

saddle

handlebars

pedals

- Listen for rattles – in a 45-minute class this can be very annoying!
- Ensure that it can easily be moved or dismantled, which may be important if you are planning to take it elsewhere.

Fig. 2.3	Handlebar adjustment point

- Remember that you get what you pay for!
- Check that the bike package comes with instructor training, which must be at least 2 days' training with certification. The Schwinn Fitness Academy (www.sfa-news.com) runs one of the most widely recognised training programmes.

Equipment

Unlike outdoor cycling, studio cycling does not entail that you have to spend a fortune on equipment. In theory you can turn up and do a class in t-shirt, shorts and trainers. However, if you want to ensure that you have a comfortable ride you would be advised to purchase at least a pair of cycling shorts.

Shorts

Cycling shorts, which are designed to be worn without underwear, have a soft liner in the

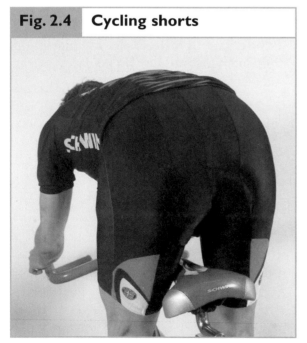

| Fig. 2.4 | **Cycling shorts** |

crotch that doesn't bunch up on a saddle the way cotton or nylon running shorts do. New liners feature antibacterial chemicals to reduce the risk of developing saddle sores. The antibacterial treatment lasts from approximately 50 to 100 washings. Lycra shorts paraded by competitive cyclists don't appeal to everyone because they don't hide anything. Clothing manufacturers such as Giordana, Nike and Oakley, to mention a few, also make baggy cycling shorts made of other lightweight fabrics with a form-fitted liner. Baggy shorts are popular among mountain bikers and tourists who may want to get off their bicycles to explore, but can also be used by a studio cyclist. These shorts can be purchased inexpensively from any local cycling shop.

Shoes

You may have seen road cyclists wearing funny-looking shoes, resembling back-to-front high heels! These shoes clip onto what known as clipless or mountain bike pedals, or often as SPDs (see Fig. 2.5). (Up until the mid-1980s cyclists used to be seen with toe clips; these are still widely used in the studio-cycling world because they are easy to use and are compatible

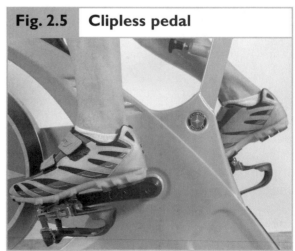

| Fig. 2.5 | **Clipless pedal** |

with any trainer and suitable for newcomers to cycling who may not feel comfortable clicking their feet into the pedals.) So why do we use clipless pedals? The shoe system features a stiff sole and firm connection to the pedal. This combination enables the cyclist to deliver leg power efficiently to the pedals. Styled after ski bindings, the sole of the shoe attaches to the pedal with a cleat that snaps firmly into place yet releases with a twist of the ankle. The soles of the shoes vary in material. Carbon-soled shoes are among some of the best due to the stiffness of the sole, ensuring no pedal power is lost; however, for studio cycling mountain-bike shoes with an SPD fitting are probably the cheapest option and most user-friendly. However, not all studio-cycling bikes have clipless pedals and if your gym doesn't you can let them know that double-sided pedals (one side with SPD fitting and the other with toe clips) can be purchased inexpensively from any local bike shop. Once you have ridden with clipless pedals you will never want to go back to using trainers – so much power and energy is wasted in the flexibility of sports shoes.

Towel and water

This may seem a rather strange thing to remind you to bring but you would be surprised at the number of people that turn up to a class without either! Cycling indoors makes you sweat a lot and it is very uncomfortable to have sweat dripping down your face and not be able to wipe it off. Another reason for bringing a towel is safety; laying the towel across the handlebars will stop your hands from slipping. A final reason is that it will stop your sweat from dripping onto the flywheel – this is especially important if it is your own bike. Human sweat is extremely corrosive and it only takes a few months for it to rust the bike.

Dehydration is something that we all neglect;

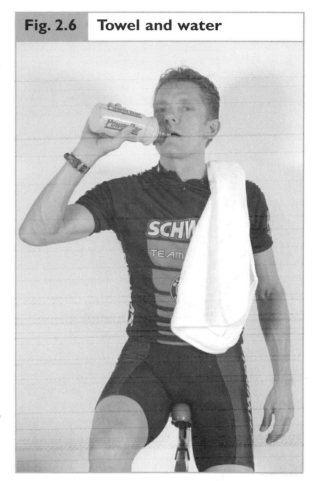

Fig. 2.6   Towel and water

most people are lacking fluid even before exercise. It is important to drink plenty of water or energy drink at regular intervals during a class. Do not wait for the instructor or coach to stop, but try to get used to drinking while you are riding; it is far easier to stay hydrated than to rehydrate yourself.

Heart rate monitor

This useful tool (see Fig. 2.7) is not essential but will help you to gauge the intensity at which you work and it is also a way to measure improved fitness, which can be a fantastic motivator. We will talk much more about heart

Fig. 2.7	Attaching a heart rate monitor

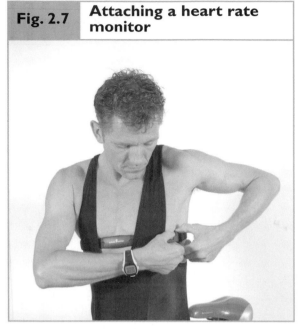

rate monitoring and its importance later on in the book in the Chapter 4, Heart Zone Training® for Studio Cycling.

Safety

Indoor cycling can be dangerous if people just get onto bikes and start pedalling. It is important always to ask your instructor before climbing aboard, or as an instructor to take control. Don't let anyone on the bike until you have explained the flywheel and braking system.

Medical history and fitness programme

An important part of being an instructor is finding out your client's medical history; if a client has a history of ill health, he or she should have a GP's permission before beginning studio cycling.

Instructor tips:

- Ensure a responsible position: be safe, knowledgeable and confident.
- Take control – it is imperative that the group understands that you, as the coach, are in control. It is your job to keep attention focused on you from the very start to ensure a safe class.
- Whether you are participating in or taking the class, it is important to make the following checks:
  - 🚴 Area check – Make sure the teaching area is free from power cables, kit bags and clothing to reduce accidents.
  - 🚴 Bikes – Although it may not be your job to maintain the bikes it is important that they are clean, working properly and ready for use.
- Spend time with the people in your class; learn at least one thing about each one, even if it is only their name! Constantly help people and offer advice.
- Cultivate a trainers' eye: look for poor technique, visual feedback, coaching points.

Note: Most health and fitness clubs will have screened their members thoroughly and will have full records; but don't get caught out, it is still up to the instructor to ask if there are any current injuries or other reasons why someone shouldn't take part in vigorous exercise. If unsure use the questionnaire below (see Fig. 2.8) for ideas to compile a simple form that covers the most important questions to ask about someone's health and fitness.

Medical questionnaire

All studio-cycling instructors must ensure their class members have completed a medical questionnaire and disclaimer, whether it is from the fitness club or to participate in the class.

There are four factors that will decide the effectiveness of the medical questionnaire.

1 What questions are asked?
2 Have they been answered correctly?
3 Is there anything that the instructor should pay attention to?

4 Does the instructor understand the answers and can he/she react to the answer if necessary?

An example of a Medical Questionnaire is shown in Figure 2.8.

Fig. 2.8 **Medical Questionnaire**	
Please complete this form and bring it with you to your class. Also bring with you towels and water, comfortable exercise clothing. Bike shorts with a pad are recommended.	

Medical History	**Yes/No**
Do you or any members of your family have past or present heart problems, i.e. heart attacks, angina, strokes or major operations?	
Are you or have you been on any long-term medication?	
If the answer to above is 'yes' please state the medication	
Do you have high blood pressure or a history of it?	
Do you suffer from asthma or shortness of breath?	
Are you a diabetic?	
Do you smoke or have you ever done so?	
Do you have epilepsy?	
Do you have any current injuries that may affect your participation in studio cycling?	
Are you pregnant?	
Do you exercise on a regular basis, i.e. 2–3 times a week for 30 mins or more?	
Is there any reason that you know of that would prevent you from exercising safely?	

If the answer to any of the above questions is 'yes' please provide more information in the box below:

Fig. 2.9 Bones and joints used in cycling

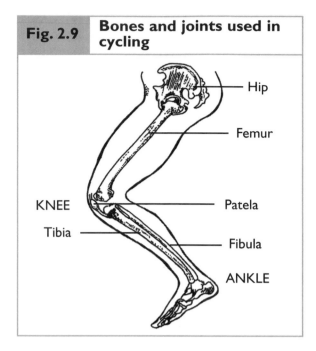

Fig. 2.10 Muscles used in cycling

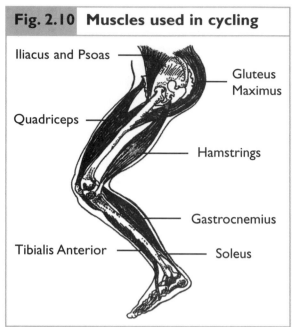

Table 2.1	Muscles of the leg and their functions	
Name	Well-known nickname	Job function
Gluteus maximus	Backside/buttocks	Seated in far back position, used with hamstrings
Biceps femoris	Hamstring	Knee flexion (heel towards buttocks), hip extension and pull-back phase
Iliacus and Psoas	Hip flexor	Hip flexion
Vastus lateralis		Recovery and push phase
Gastrocnemius	Upper calf	Plantarflexion (pointing toes), for climbing and pulling up with high resistance
Soleus	Lower calf	The calves also contribute to knee flexion
Semimembranosus		Pull-back phase
Rectus femoris		Recovery phase
Vastus medialis	Quadricep	Extension of knee and hip flexion Initial forward and down phase Transfers power to the calf muscle
Semitendinous		Pull-back phase
TA – Tibialis anterior	Shin area	Dorsiflexion (bringing foot towards shin)

Injury

If a participant is clearly injured then the coach shouldn't let them get on a bike. The coach or instructor should be visually aware. Remember that some things must be kept confidential, i.e. heart attacks, asthma and pregnancies.

It is most important that if you are planning on becoming an instructor you should purchase your own insurance, which should include instructor liability and negligence.

Anatomy and physiology

Anatomy

To understand how the leg functions we can think of it as a rigid, three-link system (the bones – see Fig 2.9). The main bone is the thighbone or femur; this is the largest bone in the body and creates rigidity for the whole leg. At the upper end of this bone it connects to the hip joint and at the lower end to the knee joint, which allows the lower part of the leg to pivot around the thigh. The strength of the lower leg is provided by two bones, the tibia and fibula. The foot connects around the lower part of these bones.

The muscles are attached to the bone by strong tendons that can control the force of the muscle to generate movement through the joints.

Most of the muscular training effect of cycling will occur in the lower body. You can see in Figure 2.10 and the muscle recruitment table (Table 2.1) the different muscles that are used in the legs at each point of the pedal revolution. There are other parts in the upper body that will be used for balance and posture and these are pinpointed in Figure 2.11. It is useful for the instructor to become familiar with these muscles and understand how they work during cycling action.

Pedal action

As force is applied to the pedals there is a physiological response that shortens or contracts the muscles moving the bones towards each other. This is known as a concentric contraction. As the muscle shortens the movement is caused. An example of this would be climbing stairs: the hip flexors lift the leg up and the quadriceps work against external

Fig. 2.11 Upper body muscles when riding a bike

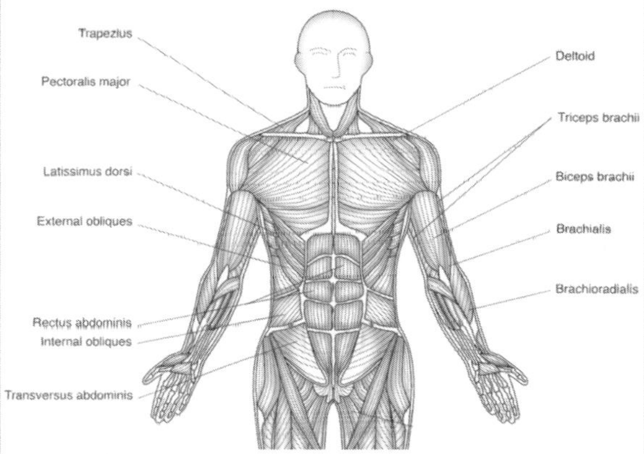

Trapezius
Pectoralis major
Latissimus dorsi
External obliques
Rectus abdominis
Internal obliques
Transversus abdominis
Deltoid
Triceps brachii
Biceps brachii
Brachialis
Brachioradialis

forces thus working concentrically. When stepping back off the step the quadriceps are working eccentrically. This means that the same muscle is capable of lengthening under external

Instructor tip:

When instructing a class don't always use the technical name for muscle; try to refer to the area of the body or the nickname. Teach the class to put their hands on the particular area and explore the feel of the muscle while pedalling slowly with good resistance.

forces or eccentric contractions.

One of the advantages that cycling has over other exercises is that the frame of the bike supports the body. The muscles are not working against gravity therefore there are only concentric contractions.

The upper body muscles will be used for support and posture (see Fig. 2.11).

Physiology

Very simply, to get the energy we need to cycle we must breathe in oxygen, which is transported to the muscles where it is combined with food (fuel). The muscle can then contract, which produces movement and force.

There is only a limited amount of fuel stored in the muscles to aid with contraction, so they rely on blood flow to supply adequate amounts of fuel as required. Cells depend on a chemical compound called adenosine triphosphate (ATP) for their immediate energy source. When ATP is broken down by chemical action into adenosine diphosphate (ADP), energy is released. The body creates ATP in two ways: by aerobic metabolism (with oxygen) and anaerobic metabolism (without oxygen).

Aerobic metabolism

Oxygen is used to manufacture ATP from fats, carbohydrates and small amounts of proteins. The by-product of this metabolism is carbon dioxide (CO_2) and water (H_2O). Carbon dioxide is diffused into the bloodstream, then carried to the lungs and exhaled. Water is given out by the body when breathing but also with increased sweating to cool the body during exercise, which is known as thermoregulation.

This system is extremely efficient, as the aerobic metabolism has no by-products to cause fatigue. So as long as the fuel is kept topped up the body can continue to produce sizeable and sustained amounts of energy for a long time.

Anaerobic metabolism

There are two forms of anaerobic metabolism (see Fig. 2.12):

1 ATP - PC system (PC = Phosphocreatine)
2 Lactic acid system

Phosphocreatine is a substance in the cell used to synthesise ATP. Stored in the muscle or produced quickly by the body for explosive power such as sprints and short extreme and powerful efforts. The duration of the energy that this system can create is only about 15 seconds.

During high-intensity efforts the muscles can produce energy when the cardiovascular system is unable to deliver sufficient oxygen to the cells to meet their demand; at this point the lactic acid system takes over. This system is also known as anaerobic glycolysis. Lactic acid is a by-product of this system and as it builds up in the muscles and bloodstream it leaves a sore or burning feeling, and results in fatigue and slowing down, creating a stress hormone response.

Initial response to exercise is for ATP stores to be utilised and then form PC, but depending on the duration of the exercise most energy will come from the aerobic energy system. This means fat metabolism for low to medium intensity and glucose for higher intensities while oxygen is present, after this no extra fat will be utilised.

In our studio-cycling programme we find a useful relationship between the heart zone percentages, cycling techniques and the current programme an instructor wishes individuals to follow. The amount of time spent on each effort is relative to the individual response and performance for any given technique. This will change as the programme develops and within each part of the programme such as warm-up, pre-main set, main set and recovery.

You can carry out each technique with a different energy system depending on

Fig. 2.12 Energy systems and metabolism

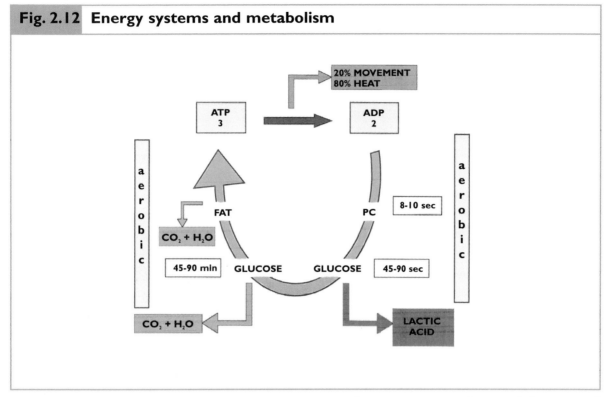

programme requirements.

For example, here are *six class variables*: 1. techniques; 2. leg speeds; 3. resistances; 4. durations; 5. energy systems; and, probably more important than all the others, 6. recovery. This will show you how important it is to plan your class programme and know exactly which variable you will choose at which point of the class. In the 'Class Profiles' later on you can see how the variables might be used, in order to help you start planning your own classes.

Examples:

1 A seated flat at 90, 100 or 110 rpm can use aerobic energy or aerobic and lactic energy or just lactic energy.

2 A standing flat at 80, 90, 100 or 110 rpm can use aerobic energy, aerobic and lactic acid energy or just lactic acid energy.

3 A seated climb at 60, 70, 80 rpm can use aerobic energy, aerobic and lactic acid energy or just lactic acid energy

4 A sprinting at 110 rpm max. can use lactic acid energy.

The key for an instructor is to choose which of the six variables you wish to focus on at each point in the class and decide how you can use them to train the individuals in the group. Knowledge, skill, understanding and empathy is required – in fact all the skills of a coach. Coaching your group will be just as much an art form as a science. When you write your class programmes start to put in the *six class variables* to jog your memory and ensure you use the correct energy systems. Each individual will respond differently to any of the variables, you will need to find out how to get the most out of each person with the different variables (see the section on 'feedbacks' to help you with this).

'Anatomy' and 'physiology' can often be overlooked in simple training terms, when in reality our body's genetic make-up is what allows us to train in the first place. While it is not vital to know the technical name for every bone and muscle it is important to know what certain muscles do and how they adapt to different forms of exercise. Studio-cycling classes can help individuals to learn more about their muscles just by allowing each class member to focus on a specific muscle and to feel it work, incorporating biomechanics at the same time (although, as we have mentioned above, it is important not to blind people with science: use the nicknames of the muscles or simply refer to the appropriate area). While the muscles are busy working so are the internal functions of the body; different types of classes, i.e. varying techniques, leg speeds, resistances, durations and energy systems, allow a class member to learn and discover exactly how the body uses oxygen and also how the metabolic rate alters when exercising. The more people learn the more they want to know; fit and healthy people want to discover more about how their bodies work so that they know that their fitness levels and general health are improving.

Instructor tips:

- Ask beginners to arrive 15 minutes before class.
- Remember beginners are often lacking in confidence and knowledge and have no idea what to expect.
- Take account of individual needs – weight loss, sporting, social etc.

The bike

If you are new to studio cycling you may not be aware of how to set your bike up correctly. It is imperative that you ask your instructor for help, because what seems to be the correct position can often leave you feeling uncomfortable after the first few minutes, fail to allow you to reach your full potential on the bike and might even lead to injury.

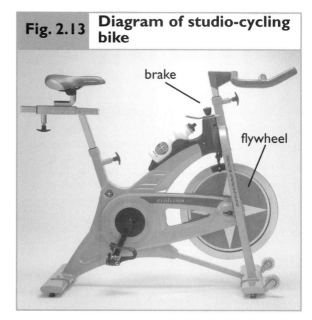

Fig. 2.13 Diagram of studio-cycling bike

brake

flywheel

The flywheel

This heavy wheel is attached to the pedals by means of a fixed gear, which means that, having begun pedalling you will not be able to stop without applying the brake or adding resistance. A professional instructor will ensure that all beginners take hold of the flywheel and move it backwards and forwards; they may then ask them to take hold of a pedal and slowly turn it making sure that no hands or fingers are in the way. If they were then asked to stop the pedals by hand, they will realise the weight of the wheel. This will help a beginner to understand the difference between a studio-cycling bike and an ordinary road bike.

The brake

The braking system on a studio bike is the simplest and most effective. While the pedals are turning the heavy flywheel is rotating at speed. To add resistance or slow the flywheel the adjustment dial is turned towards the plus sign, in an emergency the whole dial unit can be pushed or pulled towards the rider and the flywheel will stop immediately. The location and movement of this adjustment will vary from bike to bike.

The application of the flywheel and the fixed gear system is the first thing an instructor must tell a new client. Once they understand how it works, beginners can start to enjoy the benefits of a mind and body work-out

Full bike check

The instructor must check that all the bikes are fully operational and safe to sit on.

Bike maintenance

Why is maintenance so important? The answer is simple: if a bike does not function properly, whether you own it or not, it will undoubtedly disrupt your class or your own work-out. That is why it is vital that the person responsible should check all the bikes before each class and that a regular maintenance schedule is followed (see below). A brief check before the class will pick up any major faults, as will class feedback at the end of a session.

The studio-cycling bike

There are many different manufacturers of studio-cycling bikes; make sure you keep in contact with your supplier and check that he/she has basic spares in stock.

Check the following:

- Brakes
  Ensure that when the pedals are going fast the brakes stop the flywheel immediately. Depending on the braking system, the dial (calliper or brake pressure) or lever (cables) may need adjustment.
- Tensions
  Check tightness of pedals, cranks, seat, bottle cage and all screws, knobs, etc.
- Working order
  Check that the saddles move forwards and back, seat posts move up and down, handlebars move up and down, pedals rotate smoothly (no lateral movement), brakes function quickly, resistance adjustment knobs work smoothly, all pins can be pulled out and released.
- Cleanliness
  It is vital that you or your clients sit on a clean studio-cycling bike!
  Sweat is *the* most corrosive element and left on the bike will compromise every bike's performance. Dirty bikes must be cleaned by the person that rode them – or the instructor!!

Maintenance schedule

- Pre- and post-class + daily check and class records
  Check cleanliness, rust, flywheel alignment, seat position.
  Before and after each class ensure tension is off, this promotes the life of the bikes and prevents unnecessary wear. Make sure there are sufficient cleaning agents around i.e. antiseptic cleaning sprays and paper towels for class members.
- Weekly maintenance
  Drive chains – check tension and clean, lubricate, etc. Check pedals for wear on toe clips and bearings. Check drive belts, chains, etc; for exact tension or lubricants always

follow the manufacturer's specifications. Some brake pads will need soaking with a Teflon-coated silicon spray lubricant.

Ideally bikes should be fully serviced in the following way:

1–6 months
- ⚙ Replace the chain belt.
- ⚙ Reposition the flywheel.
- ⚙ Breakdown the bike, clean and lubricate.
- ⚙ Change any static positions of the bike to allow for more periodical wear of all the bikes.
- ⚙ Replace bearings. Refer to specific manufacturer manual if experiencing further difficulties.

Potential problems (**P**) and solutions (**S**):

P. You feel a jarring from the pedal: this could be a slack chain.
S. Adjustment of the flywheel will take out the slack from the chain.

P. There is no resistance on the flywheel.
S. On belt-resistance bikes the belt can work loose. Unwind the resistance dial and tighten the belt. With calliper brakes, hold in the brakes and adjust more tension against the callipers.

P. Pedals and cranks wobble laterally.
S. Tighten crank arm or tighten/replace bottom bracket bearings.

P. Bike wobbles on uneven floor.
S. Most bikes will have adjustable feet, check which side needs adjusting. There may be a locking nut, so have a spanner to fit.

P. Toe-clip straps have come out and are fraying.
S. Replace toe-clip strap, loop through the pedal with the buckle facing out, twist the strap after it has gone through the first pedal frame hole (helps to reduce strap slipping), press the

buckle together, thread the strap over the roller and under the jagged edge. There is no need to thread through the rest of the buckle.

P. Saddle is tilted at the wrong angle.
S. Undo the securing nut under the saddle and adjust saddle into horizontal position; the nose of the saddle will be slightly higher than the back.

P. Brakes vibrate or squeak.
S. Some brake pads need soaking in lubricant. Ensure it is a silicon spray with Teflon and soak the pad completely before replacing. In emergencies during the class it can be applied from the rider side as the flywheel is rotating.

On some other bikes there are inherent problems with the brakes; ensure you receive good back up from manufacturer or distributor. If you have doubts, obtain a maintenance contract with them prior to purchase. Your warranty on the frame and most parts should not be affected.

Rules

- ⚙ Never leave bike maintenance until later. Do it yourself with the knowledge and experience you have or get it done by your maintenance department now!
- ⚙ Ensure there is always a complete toolkit available near the bikes in case adjustments need to be made during your work-out or a class. Ideally you should ensure a toolkit comes with the bikes when they are purchased. Some manufacturers sell a professional bike mechanics kit which will include every tool needed to maintain and overhaul the bikes completely.
- ⚙ Use the booking system to help pinpoint bike breakdown during or after each class.

Table. 2.2	Class booking form and bike maintenance record		
Bike Number	Name	Contact No	Maintenance work to be done
1			
2			
3			
4			
5			
6			
7			
8			
9			
10			
11			
12			
13			
14			
15			
16			
17			
18			

Bike set-up

The Quick Fit

Getting a newcomer set up correctly on a bike can be a lengthy process and is not always the most viable option especially if a class is about to begin. That is why we have developed something known as the 'Quick Fit'. It is not the most accurate of measurements and can if taught incorrectly lead to confusion.

Watch your instructor or coach teach from his or her bike. If you are learning to be an instructor remember always to teach from your own bike – if you were to set up everyone individually you would never start the class!

Instructor note:
- Tuck shoe laces out of the way before you pedal.
- When all checks are being made ensure participants are sitting towards the rear of the saddle on their 'sit bones' and that they have the balls of their feet over the middle of the pedal regardless of the size of the foot in the toe clip.

Saddle height

There are three checks you must remember before starting to pedal:

- Stand on the back bar of the bike; your hip joint and hipbone will be near the top of the centre of the saddle (see Figs. 2.14 and 2.15). This will get the saddle close, but not accurate.
- Sit on the saddle with both feet on the pedals; ensure there is a slight bend in the knee when one pedal (same side) is at its lowest point.
- Set the pedals at 6 and 12 o'clock (see Fig. 2.16).
- Take the foot at 6 o'clock off and **scrape the heel** across the pedal from outside in (see Fig. 2.17).
- Adjust height if too low or too high (see Fig. 2.18). Your 6 o'clock leg must be straight and hips level. When the ball of the foot is placed on the pedal this will give the 'slight' bend in the knee (see Fig. 2.19).
- Sit to the rear of the saddle ensuring both feet are locked into the pedals; when rotating slowly there should be no rocking of the hips.

Saddle position (fore and aft)

The fore and aft position is a facility that not all studio cycling bike manufacturers have taken into account when making the bike. However most leading brands such as Schwinn do allow you to alter the saddle position.

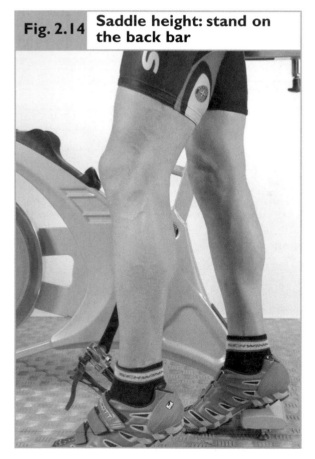

Fig. 2.14 Saddle height: stand on the back bar

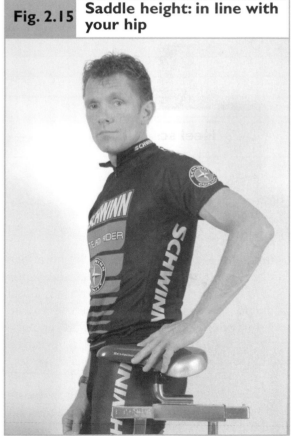

Fig. 2.15 Saddle height: in line with your hip

Fig. 2.16 Pedals at 6 and 12 o'clock

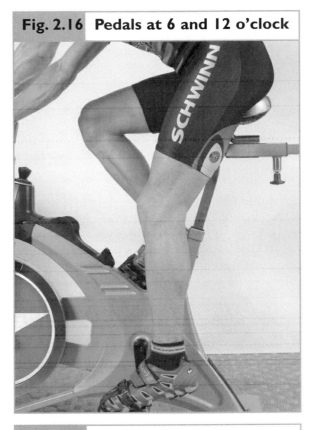

Fig. 2.19 Slight bend in the knee

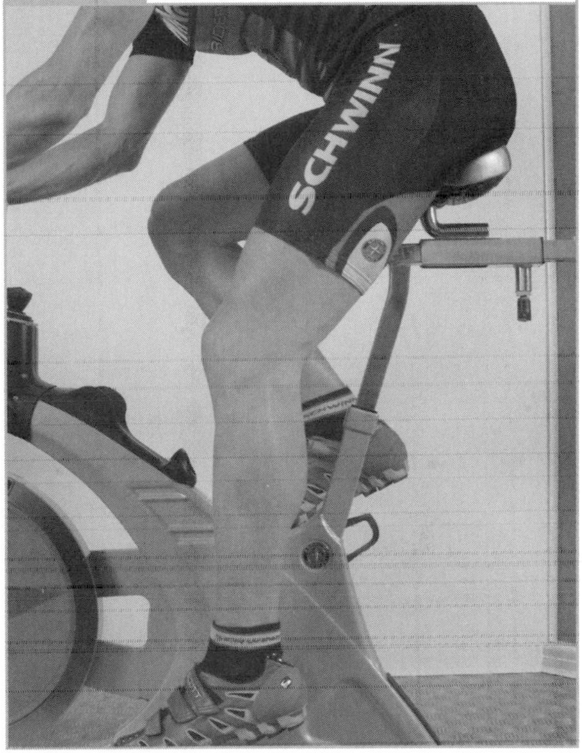

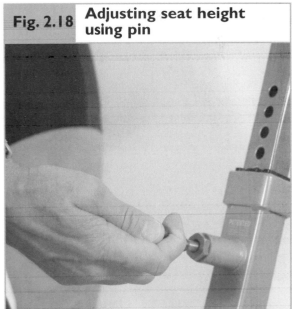

Fig. 2.17 Heel scrape

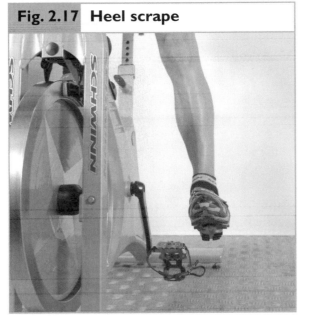

Fig. 2.18 Adjusting seat height using pin

Rules

- ✦ It is better for the saddle to be too low than too high as you will have already set the saddle to hip height so you will not be too low. Also bikes with pin system adjustments would be better with the pin in the hole below rather than the one above.
- ✦ Try and remember your positions. Many bikes have numbers listed on the adjustments; write them down and carry them in your kitbag so that you don't have to ask again.
- ✦ If you are not sure about your position ask your instructor to watch you pedal. The position your instructor places you in may seem rather alien at first but once you have been to a few classes you will begin to get used to it; if you are still uncomfortable alter your position – there is no real right or wrong.

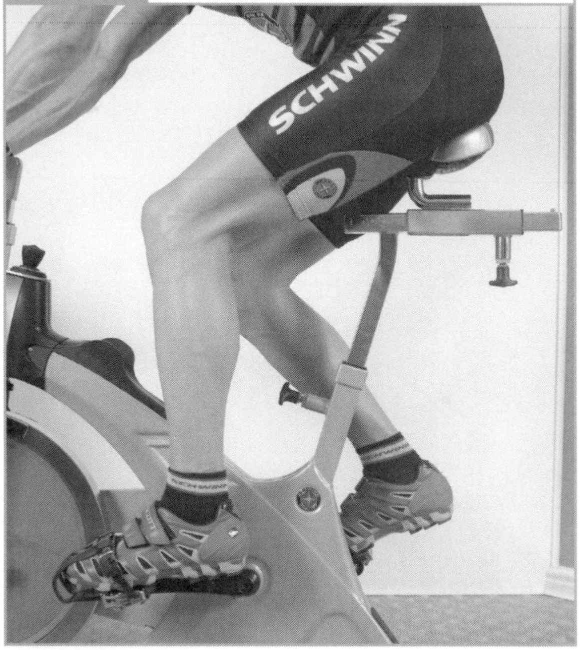

Instructor tips:

- • When explaining each set-up position, get off your bike and make an adjustment to it even if it doesn't need it. Beginners are often very self-conscious and if they see you making an adjustment to your bike it encourages them to do the same. If a beginner left their saddle a bit too high it will be very uncomfortable by the end of a class!
- • Show the set-up on both sides so that all the class members can see.

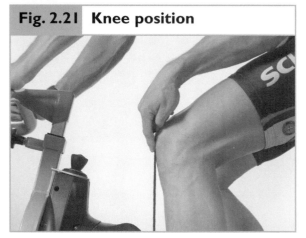

Fig. 2.20 Pedals at 3 and 9 o'clock position

Fig. 2.21 Knee position

It is important that you sit towards the back of the saddle with the balls of your feet placed in the middle of the pedal. The next step is to move the feet to 3 and 9 o'clock positions (see Fig. 2.20), then add some resistance to keep the foot position in the same place. Lean your body forwards, remembering to keep your back as straight as possible, and look down directly above the kneecap of the front leg. Just below the kneecap draw an imaginary line through the middle part of the pedal or very slightly back (see Fig. 2.21). If the line passes in front of the middle pedal the seat needs to be adjusted back slightly and vice versa. Remember that when a seat position is moved back it can increase the saddle height, so this may need to be adjusted again. Cyclists who specialise in triathlon and time trials often have their own preference for saddle positions.

Instructor tip:

Your front foot, when placed at 3 o'clock, should be at the same angle as when you are pedalling. Correct this by pedalling a few rotations without resistance and find your natural position.

Handlebar height

As a general rule the handlebars should be level with or below the seat, and for newcomers to cycling slightly higher (see Fig. 2.22). You will find that as you become more flexible you should be able gradually to lower your handlebars (see Fig. 2.23). This aerodynamic position is beneficial allowing you to feel more

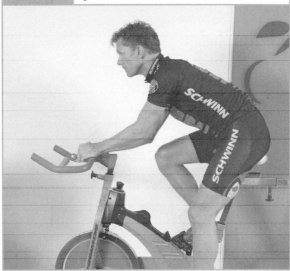

Fig. 2.23 Aerodynamic handlebar position

and more like an outdoor cyclist; however, there are exceptions, such as people with poor flexibility of the lower back who may wish to have their handlebars a bit higher. If you do suffer from back problems then a slightly higher handlebar position is encouraged initially, but progressively lowering over a period of time will help mobility providing this does not aggravate the injury.

Your goal is to attempt to get your handlebar height as low as possible. Time trialists or triathletes can often be seen crouched in an

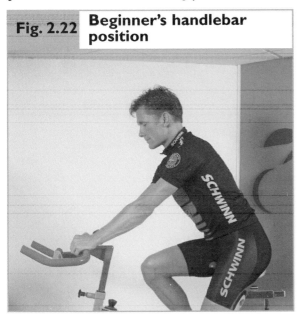

Fig. 2.22 Beginner's handlebar position

Instructor tip:

Look at all the bikes before the class. If all the handlebars are set too high the instructor before you has not applied this principle and the class may have felt pressure in the crutch. During a period of gradually lowering handlebars make sure a correct stretch regime is completed to reach the major muscle groups: gluteus maximus, hamstrings and hip flexors must be thoroughly stretched and lengthened. See p.81 for further information on stretching.

aerodynamic position on their aerobars. Other than just looking and feeling like a cyclist you will also notice that the higher the handlebars the more heavily the rider sits in the saddle. With poor biomechanics this can add to crutch discomfort.

Handlebar fore and aft

Again, as we mentioned in the section on saddle position, not all bikes have fore and aft adjustment for the handlebars. Where provided, it is used to improve comfort when riding.

- Sit up and let your arms hang by your side, allow them to bend naturally do not straighten them like you are in the army, let them hang loosely. They will hang with an angle of 15–21 degrees.
- Reach forwards with the natural bend still in the elbows and take hold of the handlebars, with the arms relaxed there should be a right angle (90 degrees) between the upper arm and torso. If the angle is more than a right angle the handlebars are too far forward and vice versa. If the bike doesn't have this option and you feel uncomfortable just resting your hands on the bars, slide them further out until you get the correct angle.

Instructor tip:

This is a good opportunity to get the group to acknowledge the person next to them; it can be difficult to check your own right angle. Again this is an adjustment people often neglect so get off your bike and alter your position to encourage clients to do the same

Scientific set-up

This is the most accurate way of setting someone up on a bike; however, it is not as quick and easy as the method above. So why do

Instructor tip:

It is advisable that when changing a set-up position using the goniometer an adjustment of no more than 5° angle should be made at one time thus allowing the body to get used to a small angle change first.

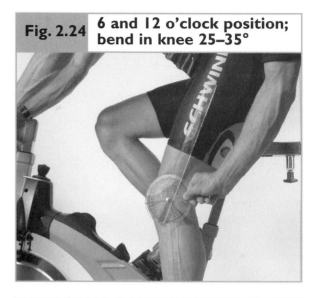

Fig. 2.24 **6 and 12 o'clock position; bend in knee 25–35°**

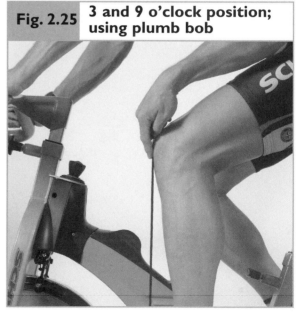

Fig. 2.25 **3 and 9 o'clock position; using plumb bob**

Fig. 2.26 | **Bend in arm 15–21°**

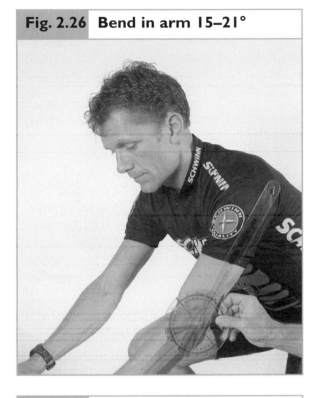

Fig. 2.27 | **Angle of upper arm and torso 89–90°**

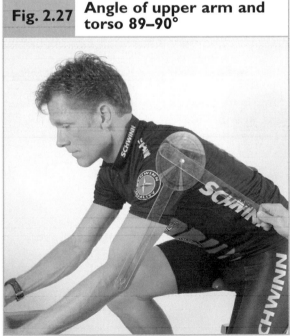

we need to do a scientific set-up if we can use the Quick Fit? This method can be used if somebody has a health concern after they have been studio cycling a few times and are still unable to gain optimum comfort. Many instructors have found that this method shows professionalism; the person with the injury may find this of psychological help; the majority of the time they already have the exact position but just need reassurance. A professional instructor will use a tool called a goniometer to measure correct angles of deflection in the knee and torso and a plumb bob to measure the knee position over the pedal.

- 6–12 o'clock. Bend in knee = 25–35° (see Fig. 2.24)
- 3-9 o'clock. Front knee, bottom of knee cap (with plumb bob) (see Fig. 2.25)
- Bend in arms = 15–21° (see Fig. 2.26)
- Upper arm and torso = 89–90° (see Fig. 2.27)

Important considerations for body position and injury prevention

- Force is channelled into the pedals with or without resistance, with no unnecessary movement unless upper body movements have been incorporated for variety or balanced training.
- A relaxed position with slightly bent elbows as well as relaxed neck and shoulders will promote comfort and allow you to work at the desired level.
- Your goal is to get comfortable enough to be in a road cyclist's aerodynamic tuck position – low upper body, bent elbows, and stretched out position with the seat pushed back. An instructor who looks natural in this position is leading by example.
- Your knees should be very slightly angled inwards to reduce the pressure laterally.
- Hands and wrists must stay straight, loose

Fig. 2.28 | Knee position

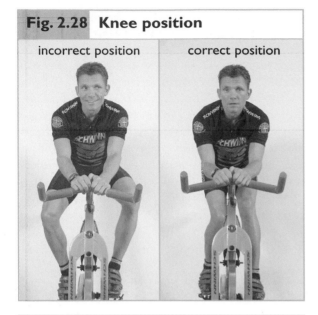

incorrect position   correct position

Fig. 2.29 | Wrist position

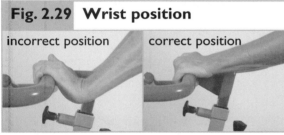

incorrect position   correct position

Instructor tip:

You need to ensure you coach the class member: ask their medical background, find out their goals. Most importantly of all, learn the above technical aspects of studio cycling; it would look unprofessional if you were faced with a straightforward question that you were unable to answer. There are further considerations for cyclists and triathletes that need understanding. For example, why a triathletes saddle is further forward than a road cyclist's, and what the optimum position for the cleat on a cycling shoe is with different types of cyclists. If you don't know all the answers it is your job to find out and be professional.

and relaxed. Gripping the bars tightly increases tension throughout the whole body.

Studio-cycling techniques

Biomechanics (pedalling technique)

The biomechanics are perhaps the most important part of cycling. Professional cyclists spend 90% of their training time practising their pedalling technique; it can improve strength and even prevent injury. When training professionals are constantly trying to improve their feel and comfort during the pedal stroke. We must build this into every one of our classes to help the clients forget about the bike and get on with getting fit!

Six points to why biomechanics are so important:

1 To improve muscle balance
2 To reduce muscle injury
3 To improve pedalling efficiency
4 To aid recovery
5 To increase comfort in the saddle
6 To help relaxation of the upper body.

There are four parts to successful biomechanics; they are simple and easy to teach if you coach them during the class using basic easy-to-understand coaching points. When the four parts are put together it is possible to apply pressure throughout the 360° pedal stroke – remember, practice makes perfect!

The pedal stroke

Correct biomechanics of the pedal stroke requires practise and accuracy. Fixed gearing (as with studio-cycling bikes) creates a continuous movement (you may have seen the track cycling during the Olympics, the bikes used for those events work similarly to a studio-cycling bike in that they have a fixed wheel, there is no brake.)

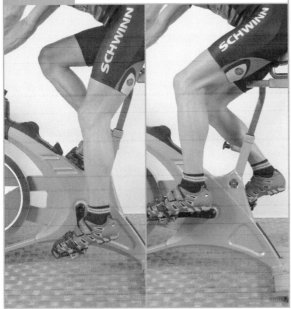

Fig. 2.30 Pedal stroke: forward and down motion

Fig. 2.31 Pedal stroke: backward and upward position

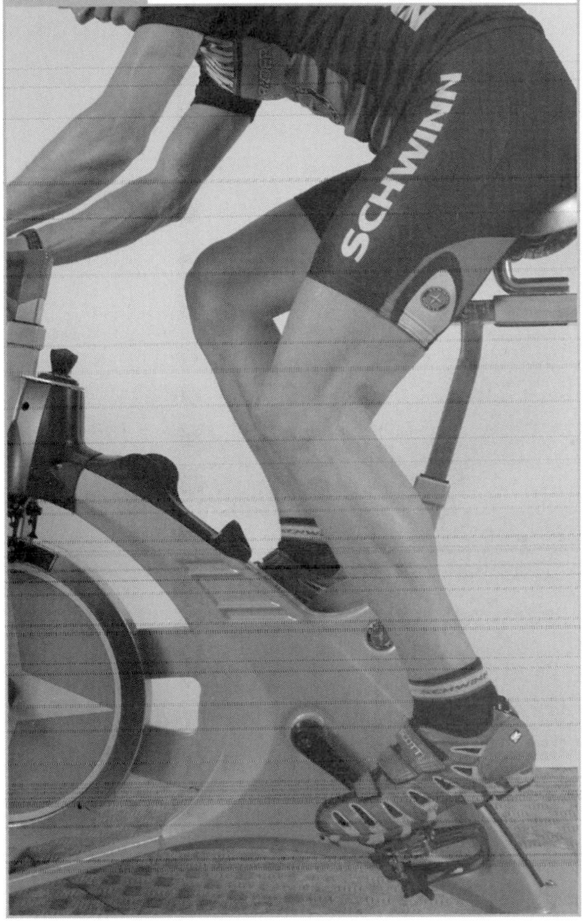

Instructor says:

'Throw your shins forwards' or 'push your toes into the ends of your shoes' or 'push forwards.'

Instructor says:

'Push down through the bottom of your shoe' or 'feel the pressure on the bottom of your foot increase', 'feel your backside become lighter in the saddle', 'and down'.

Instructor says:

'Pull your foot backwards' or 'scrape dirt from the bottom of your shoe'.

1 The pedal stroke is started by **pushing forwards** with the foot. The quadriceps and gluteus maximus muscles are active in this motion.

2 The next step is the 'power' part of the stroke. It comes from the pushing down of the pedal from the ball of the foot. The effort comes from the quadriceps group, with the gastrocnemius (calfs) active more towards the bottom of the stroke.

3 The next part comes when the foot is **pulled backwards** at the bottom of the stroke. The hamstring group of muscles are contracting during this part of the pedal stroke.

4 The last part of the pedal stroke is **pulling up**. The hamstring group of muscles and the hip flexors are responsible for this action.

25

Putting the stroke together

When we put the four parts together we can create a simple easy to remember phrase:

PUSH   FORWARDS   and   DOWN
PULL   BACK   and   UP

This action can best be described as an 'oval circle', it is done with continuous power and pressure this becomes one fluid movement, known as pedalling efficiency.

Fig. 2.32	Pattern of force through the pedal

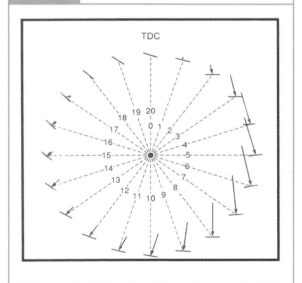

Figure 2.32 shows the pattern of force through the pedal. The pedal starts at TDC (top dead centre). The crank arm is shown as a dotted line which is moving clockwise for one revolution. The whole stroke has been divided

into measurements from 1–20. The short, bold line shows the angle of the pedal at each of the 20 measurements. The arrow shown on most of the pedals is the optimum force required at each point for maximum efficiency. If there is not enough force all the way round the rider will be less efficient and this could result in a negative training effect. Enough resistance must be on the flywheel to give the rider something to pedal against so that he/she is pedalling concentrically and not eccentrically as when someone is spinning too fast and their legs are getting pulled around. This can result in injuries, discomfort and bouncing on the saddle.

Pedalling efficiency

Goals for pedalling efficiency are set by the instructor or coach who is looking for perfect form during the full stroke which is then transferred into many strokes or rpms (revolutions per minute) or 'cadence', the cyclists' term. Cyclists spend months and years developing good pedalling efficiency at high cadence. There is, however, no correct cadence, only what feels right depending on the resistance level and suggested terrain. In studio cycling we must set some guidelines for safety, training effect and realism. These guidelines are given with the basic cycling techniques below.

Both indoors and outdoors, a cyclist can never practise pedalling technique enough. If you are having a bad day on the bike then concentrate on your technique; it will not only help you to become a better cyclist but it will make the class or ride finish quicker!

Pedal action drills:

We can devise useful drills for the class members to 'play' with:

1 Muscle initialisation: ride with focus on a particular muscle and feel it work during the full stroke. Hold this focus for at least 15

seconds then swap legs. Repeat 2–5 times. You can also build in extra time on a weak leg. Start in the saddle, but eventually you can use these drills in or out of the saddle.

2 Focus on glutes/quads – use alternate legs, let the other leg (the uninterested leg) float around.

3 Try one leg forward and down while the other leg pulls back and up, then swap over. Change the interval and do 2 or 4 one way then repeat with the opposite leg. Repeat this kind of game in every class. It is ideal as a warm-up or pre-main set. See how this technique affects the heart rate response, then use it to maintain or even raise the heart rate level as part of a set.

4 To add more 'feel' to the movement stay in the saddle and take one arm off the bar and place to the same side you are working on with the other arm. Keep the body in its usual position.

5 'Efficiency feel': Slow leg speed down to below 60 rpm, add a modicum of resistance. Explore the four different phases of the pedal action. Use muscle awareness with each individual, for example name the muscles and describe their role. You can even get the clients to touch the particular muscle as it is being used. Add the calf action to the full stroke so they can feel its power.

Handlebars and hand position

The handlebars and hand positions need to be established once you have gained an understanding of how to get yourself on the bike and how to pedal correctly. We use these positions to help to focus and to see where professional cyclists would place their hands in order to gain maximum benefit.

Position – narrow: 80–120 rpm

We use this position for seated flat cycling. Your hands are placed in a narrow position loosely

on the bars, shoulders are relaxed with a slight bend in the elbows. Wrists should always stay above the hands (see Fig. 2.33).

| Fig. 2.33 | **Narrow handlebar position** |

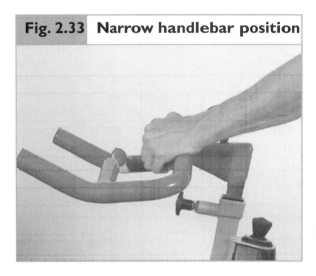

Position – wide: 60–80 rpm for hills and 80–120 for flat roads

This position can also be used for seated flats for people with broad shoulders or seated climbing as well as standing flats, combination flats (seated/standing) and the start position to combination hills (see Fig. 2.34). This is an alternative to position–narrow.

| Fig. 2.34 | **Wide handlebar position** |

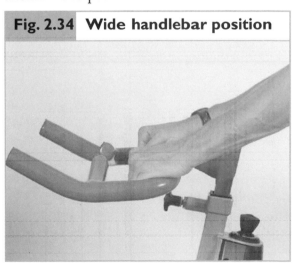

Position – narrow aerodynamic/triathlon

This position can be used for riding downhill or into a headwind. An extended arm position along the inside bars is also used for low-profile riding as with aero bars on time trial or triathlon bikes, and can be used to help with breathing if needed. The hands can grip the bars for support or rest loosely for a more relaxed grip. This position is used for triathlons, time trialing or riding into a headwind. It can be quite uncomfortable for some riders who don't have the mobility and flexibility, in which case it can be built gradually in to the programme, extending the time (see Fig. 2.35).

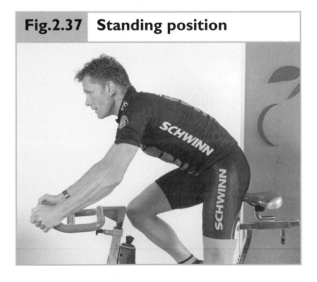

Fig. 2.35 Narrow aerodynamic position

Position – mountain bike bullhorn wide aerodynamic

This position is used by people with longer forearms and torsos as well as an advanced aerodynamic tuck position in mountain biking or on the brake hoods or drop handlebars on the road. It is an alternative position to narrow aerodynamic (see Fig. 2.36).

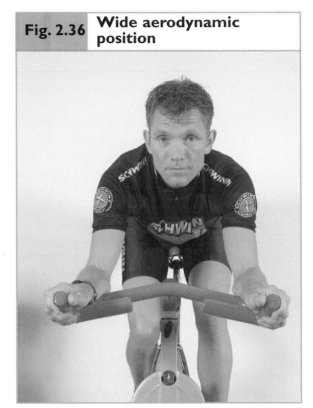

Fig. 2.36 Wide aerodynamic position

Fig.2.37 Standing position

Position – standing

Used for standing climbs (high resistance) and sprinting. The hands are gripped round the ends of the bars and the thumb comes in front of the ends. The palms are facing inwards (see Fig. 2.37).

Body positions

In studio cycling there are two basic body positions, **sitting** and **standing**. These combined with the terrain and hand positions create techniques that are similar to cycling outdoors. Once these are learnt there are many variations that can be added and used to make your journey interesting, challenging, safe, fun and effective.

Once class members have mastered sitting they should learn how to stand; it will be up to the instructor to gauge if they are ready for that and to progress to more advanced techniques.

Instructor tip:

It is good to remind the inexperienced clients or class members that they must learn the basics first. After all no one can get fit in a day, but this is their first step and pretty soon they will be amazed at the progress they have made. You need to make positive suggestions that motivate and challenge them to reach their potential. This is the start of studio-cycling coaching: see chapter on coaching.

For each technique you can use a symbol to help you plan your classes or profiles. The circle is a wheel. Inside the wheel is the type of terrain and technique. Put the wheels together to create a map. The maps become part of the 'ride profiles'.

Basic cycling techniques: signs and maps

Types of riding

Seated flat

Cadence guidelines = 80–120 rpm (revolutions per minute)

This is the easiest and most basic of positions from which we can develop all other techniques. It is possible to extend the length or time that we train in this position to develop the mind/body strength as well as stamina and endurance. It can be the hardest technique in terms of intensity, duration and high cadence – e.g. 100+ rpm (see Fig. 2.38).

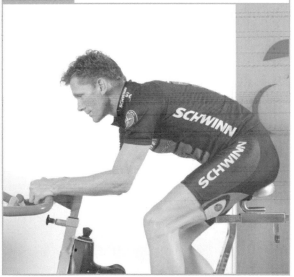

Fig. 2.38 Seated flat position

By sitting in the saddle with a controlled resistance we can rotate the pedals quickly against resistance to develop speed. The cyclist's term for this is 'spinning'. In this position we first learn to develop leg speeds (cadence) and rhythm to the music during the class. You or the instructor should choose music at the rhythm that suits the type of conditions you envisage on the road. Your feet should be in a neutral (horizontal) position.

Coaching points:

- Position your sit bones on raised or rear part of the saddle.
- Position balls of feet over middle of pedal.
- Knees should be in line over toes.
- Lengthen your spine.
- Your upper body position should bend at the hips and not by rounding the back.
- Sufficient resistance should be used to allow the body weight to be supported by legs and prevent bouncing in the saddle.
- The legs taking the weight allows upper body to relax. Arms soft, elbows in, straight wrists and loose grip on handlebars normally narrow position, drop and relax shoulders.

Seated climbs (hills and mountains)

Cadence guidelines = 60–80 rpm

As your resistance is added the cadence should get slower; the body shifts back in the saddle and a toe movement can be used to allow all the correct muscles to come into play to give optimum force against the pedals (push forwards and down, pull back and up). This activates the calf muscle and increases the force through the pedals. Cyclists should relax their upper bodies, the neck and the arms (bend the elbows); let the hands rest lightly on the bars, normally in a wide grip unless it is more comfortable to rest the arms in a narrow position (see Fig. 2.39).

Coaching points:

- Coaching points are similar to seated flat.
- It is very important to remember and focus on relaxation of the upper body.
- Experienced cyclists may try to adjust the height of the saddle downwards and slide the

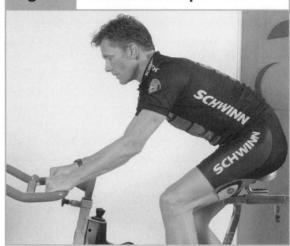

Fig. 2.39 Seated climb position

saddle back for this exercise, although moving back in the saddle is normally sufficient.

- The tempo of the music should slow down according to the class requirements; everyone will find a different beat from the same piece of music as well as finding their own hill. This is the time when you allow yourself to go and explore your own journey and rhythm.

Standing flat

Cadence guidelines = 60–100 rpm for beginners, 110+ for advanced studio cyclists

You should have certain element of resistance on the flywheel for control whilst standing on the pedals out of the saddle. Light rhythmic strokes support each revolution. Keep your upper body relaxed with the head and back in a neutral position. With arms having a very slight bend, and hands in a wide position towards the back of the handlebars (see Fig. 2.41), use the buttocks, hamstrings and quads to pump the legs freely. Your shoulders will move gently from side to side as you transfer the weight through the pedals. For advanced and more challenging technique limit your head and shoulders movement, focusing on and keeping the legs from completely straightening – the hips will be still. Your legs should be flowing in an oval movement and your hips over the bottom bracket.

Fig. 2.40 Standing flat position

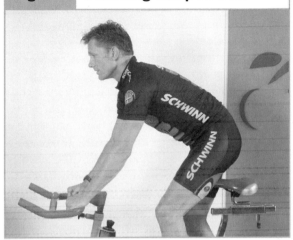

Coaching Points:

⚙ Ensure your clients have sufficient resistance before attempting to stand up – a good gauge is if it is proving challenging to pedal whilst sitting in the saddle.

⚙ Rise out of the saddle in one smooth movement.

⚙ The bottom should be just touching the tip of the saddle.

⚙ The hips should be over the centre of the bike.

⚙ The upper body should be relaxed.

⚙ The grip should be loose.

⚙ Transfer body weight through the pedals.

Standing climb

Cadence guidelines = 60–80 rpm

As the road gets steeper, the hill becomes a mountain and the air gets thinner, the instructor prepares his class for a standing climb. Your

emotive music should change as everyone in the class begins to challenge him- or herself. Gradually in one movement your backside comes off the saddle. Your bottom stays in line with the saddle, the grip is now at standing position (as mentioned above), your nose crosses the centre line with the rhythm of the music beat and your body transfers its weight through the pedals. The arms can be used to pull against the bars and power you up the mountain.

The ideal cadence can be anything from 60–80 rpm; let the rhythm of the music match the leg speed.

Fig. 2.41 Standing climb position

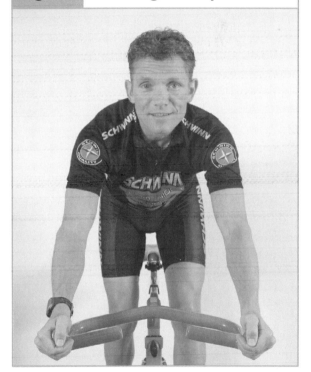

Coaching points:

⚙ Ensure your clients have sufficient resistance before attempting to stand up – a good gauge is if it is proving difficult to pedal while sitting in the saddle.

♲ Rise out of the saddle in one smooth movement.

♲ The bottom should just be touching the tip of the saddle.

♲ The hips should be over the centre of the bike.

♲ The upper body should be relaxed.

♲ The grip should be loose.

♲ Transfer body weight through the pedals.

♲ The hands should be placed in wide position at the ends of the bars.

♲ Relax your upper body.

♲ Pull lightly against the bars.

Instructor tip:

Emphasis should be placed on the correct amount of resistance; you will find it easier to pedal out of the saddle than in, if the right amount is used. If you are finding it difficult and you are struggling to stay up or find yourself leaning forwards and supporting all your weight with your arms it could mean that you do not have enough resistance on the flywheel.

Combination flats or hills

Combinations (flats or hills) are sometimes referred to as 'jumping'; it is a more advanced technique that can perform many tasks (sometimes it is necessary to challenge both instructor and class!); combinations can be performed both in and out of the saddle, on flat or hilly terrain. Be careful to ensure riders know this is *not* the hardest thing they will do on a bike (perhaps the hardest method of cycling is sitting in the saddle riding fast against resistance for a long period of time).

Moving in and out of the saddle can help you to develop timing, leg strength, muscular endurance, cardiovascular fitness and balance. Always use visualization and specific challenges like the finish of a race or jumping away from a pack. Your jumps can vary at different intervals – set the class goals depending on individual levels. It is vital to teach correct form with fluid continuous movement of the legs while lifting them both in and out of the saddle (see Fig. 2.42 and Fig. 2.43).

As you begin to develop, set challenges by coming out of the saddle with a burst of power and increasing the pedal speed – not unlike breaking away in a race.

Combinations, or jumping, is an ideal way of introducing motivational goal-setting. The clever techniques you can use will inspire both instructor and class if used at the right time. Don't use them just because you run out of things to do: use them to motivate, break up a tough set or raise the heart rate to the correct zone. For more advanced cyclists who can do this easily it is ideal to mobilise and relax them if used between main sets.

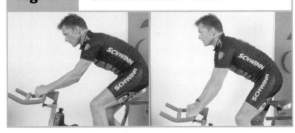

Fig. 2.42 Combination flats

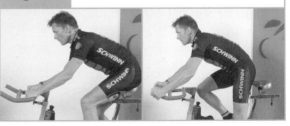

Fig. 2.43 Combination hills

Coaching points:

♲ Aim to achieve one smooth movement.

♲ Keep the hips back when out of the saddle.

♲ Never jump for less than a count of four.

Stepping

Stepping is perhaps about as rhythmically challenged as a studio cyclist can get! It can be used for a number of different reasons:

🚴 Variety.

🚴 Highlighting music rhythm.

🚴 Improving flexibility and mobility of the lower back whilst encouraging people to bend at the hip.

🚴 Encouragement of group participation.

🚴 Focusing on muscle strengths, weaknesses and balance (see advanced training chapter).

🚴 Relief after an intense effort.

🚴 Prolonging the heart rate zone work.

Different timings can be used when stepping and it is entirely up to you to come up with your own choice of music. The simplest technique is to work backwards from 8, count down to 6, then 4, and so on. The ultimate goal is to get down to single counts where you choose one leg to lead with the upper body in time with the beat of the music, and then change legs.

> **Instructor tip:**
>
> It is important that you have practised this part thoroughly before attempting it in a class, because if your timing is out it will confuse the group. Use music with a simple, distinctive beat that is easy for everyone to follow. Try and give a demonstration of what you are about to do with your stepping and when you are going to do it so people know what to expect. Remember this is a technique beyond normal cycling, although there are benefits that include muscular balancing in weaker leg muscles, development of team spirit with group uniform movements and timely increments of heart zone sets.
>
> Try a count in: 'watch me – 3, 2, 1 – and come forwards and up' etc.

Pace change – walk, jog, run and sprint

These four pace changes can be used in studio cycling, and any of them can be incorporated into the different roads we ride. Each one has a different interpretation of road riding depending on where we are on our journey. Great care must be taken when changing pace; it is imperative that technique and form are not neglected in order to do so. For example, you would not attempt pace change if you are a beginner or any of your clients are instructing them, as they are still learning the basic techniques and need to ride at their own rhythm. Although the slow walk pace may be used for reasons of technique pace change challenges are far more relevant to intermediate or advanced studio cyclists.

> **Instructor tip:**
>
> When teaching pace change give a demonstration to the group so they can follow. The terms used are not specific to cycling in order to be more familiar to most people.

Pace 1 known as 'walking pace' 60+ rpm
Walking pace is coached by pedalling below the beat of the music. It can be used during different parts of the class such as warm-up or recovery, stretching for upper body, or during a distinctive part after adding resistance. It could be useful for class members who are learning new techniques.

Pace 2 known as 'jogging pace' 80–120+ rpm
Jogging pace is coached by pedalling with the beat of the music. It can be used at all stages of the class and the intensity is determined by the type of challenge and how much resistance is added. Jogging is the most common pace during classes and generally the group will be in their aerobic zone.

Pace 3 known as 'running'

Running is coached by pedalling above the beat of the music. It is used during a more difficult challenge with resistance or even going downhill with less resistance. The technique must not be forsaken for more speed – you must use sufficient resistance to say in control.

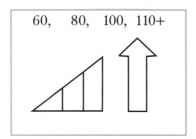

Pace 4 known as 'sprinting'

This is a very advanced technique and will be practised only after 6 weeks of consistent training in 2–3 classes a week. It can be performed both in and out of the saddle, and an instructor should be able to assess when a class is ready to start sprinting.

The music will be an upbeat sound with a fast-moving rhythm. You should increase the pace whilst developing at your own level, staying in control. If it is your first time sprinting, quickly reassess where the brake is in an emergency. You may also want to check to see if your toe clips are tight. Feet that come out of the pedal whilst moving at even low speeds are liable to get hurt because the pedals are being driven by the weight of the heavy flywheel. Sprinting in the saddle requires a relaxed upper body with no tension. There is usually challenging resistance and it is only done for a limited time period or interval of no more than 15 seconds. The resistance will be sufficient to make it very tough to pedal faster than 110 rpm.

The cadence can go from 80 to 140+ rpm. On the road this is very difficult to achieve and a new level of focus and energy output can be gained. In a class situation it helps to focus if you imagine a sudden breakaway or finish to a race. Your competitors come from behind and catch you by surprise. Add challenging resistance (change the gears), increase leg speed.

Out of the saddle a new degree of rhythm, power focus and balance will be achieved. You will have to master relaxation of the hips, neck and shoulders before you find sprinting out of the saddle comfortable. Practise is the key! This technique normally starts on an incline with good resistance. Change the gears, up the tempo and rise out of the saddle for a hill sprint of no more than 15 seconds.

Upper body movements

> **Instructor tip**:
>
> WARNING!
> In some studio-cycling programmes instructors use upper body techniques too often and overemphasise them. Please remember as a guideline that they should not be part of the main set.

There are several different upper body moves. They are only ever used to:

- Mobilise, relax and de-stress the upper body (head, neck and shoulders).
- Find the music rhythm.
- Recover and motivate yourself when the journey gets too tough.
- Group participation.
- Lower back relaxation.
- Recovery.

Rhythm presses

No upper body movements will ever be a focal point of the class. They must be simple, there is no need for extravagant complicated movements as with some forms of aerobics. Remember you are training to be a studio cyclist not an aerobic instructor.

The body dips slowly using the arms (shoulders, chest, triceps, abdominals). You should remain seated with hands in narrow or wide position. This is an advanced mobilising technique, not an arm exercise. It is used to relax the hips so that the rider can develop an aerodynamic position, find rhythm and develop leg technique by focusing on and lengthening the spine whilst repeating this exercise in the warm-up. It is not done outside on the road but within the studio, and can aid development if used at the right time. Remember: don't use this for any other reason, such as aerobics on a bike.

Abdominal work

The abdominal muscles have been known for a long time to be one of the most important areas of the body, protecting posture and the back. As in martial arts, power comes from the stomach and all techniques originate from correct tension of the lower abdomen. If you control the centre of gravity at your stomach all the techniques used in studio cycling will become easier. As you sprint or make any sudden burst of energy the abdominal muscles should be active. For more relaxed movements the stomach can be kept relaxed even when the heart rate is very high.

During some classes contraction of the stomach can be emphasised for some movements, so that a light localised muscular training effect is felt.

Breathing

Control of the breathing can enhance athletic performance, increase energy and encourage the body to relax. Correct diaphragmatic breathing will activate the parasympathetic nervous system. The tenth cranial nerve is responsible for calming and relaxation. There are two types of breathing, shallow breathing from the chest and diaphragmatic breathing, which is deep. Shallow breathing by people under pressure and stressed is ineffective, reducing mental and physical capacity. Deep breathing pulls the air into the lower lobes of the lungs where there is more blood available for oxygen exchange.

Breathing techniques:
- Breathe deeply with the diaphragm by expanding the abdomen when you inhale and contracting it when you exhale.
- During the warm-up and recovery phases of the class breathing should be in through the nose and out through the mouth.
- An advanced exercise is to ride with a steady but elevated heart rate and breathe only through the nose. This will help you to focus and control and help work the body to relax under pressure.
- Breathplay™: techniques can be used to focus the class away from the legs and heart rate and relax the mind. In advanced classes this can be employed to emphasise breathing rhythms. The training effect is gained by changing the pattern of breathing. It may help anyone who has respiratory problems to open the airways and increase respiratory efficiency before or during a class.

Studio cycling programme:
- Select a 90 rpm or bpm track (can be 180 bpm)
- Use a 6/3 at 90 rpm
  6 part breaths out – 3 part breaths in during three interval types, e.g. 5×30 seconds, 3×1 minute, 2×2 minutes.

To expand on the ideas above try to exhale with a shout, or by counting, as with countdown techniques used in fitness classes. This can have a training effect as well as opening the airways and possibly creating a light-hearted atmosphere between hard sets with an element of team building. Some clubs in America have even gone as far as to include karaoke spins, although if an instructor needs to resort to this to keep his or her class members happy, he or she hasn't interpreted this book properly! Keep the social scene for the bar after the class.

> **Instructor tip:**
>
> Make breathing noises to help you with this technique. You should experience a pressurised, hissing 6-count sound 'sss-sss-sss-sss-sss-sss' for the exhale and a 3-count relaxing sound 'aaa-aaa-aaah' for the inhale. For any who are self-conscious, these sounds do not have to be loud.
>
> Some athletes, including gold medallist cyclists, have noticed breathing benefit by trying this training. It may help class members in some useful ways and give you a new focus for the class.
>
> Source: www.breathplay.com Ian Jackson.

Health concerns

For a list of common complaints that both newcomers and advanced cyclists alike may ask an instructor's advice about, see Table 2.3. A studio-cycling instructor must be professional, have the knowledge to understand the problem and know how and where to look to help rectify it. Some of the complaints may have been experienced personally by the instructor; most of them are related to bike set-up.

If there is no apparent reason why someone stops participating in a class it may be because they are uncomfortable in some way, and usually the problem can be easily prevented. You will not have time at the beginning of the class to counsel people individually, so you should encourage them to arrive early for the next class or be willing to wait behind after the class so you can give 100 per cent of your attention to them. They will be grateful that not only are you willing to help them but you are also knowledgeable enough to give advice. This all adds to your reputation as a professional studio-cycling instructor.

The first thing you would do is to ensure that the complaint is not related to an old or outstanding injury. Often many people think that having a knee operation perhaps only four weeks ago is irrelevant and may not tell you; but this information is vital, especially if this is where the health complaint is located. There is only so much you can do to help someone; in the long run it is to some extent a matter of the person's common sense.

If there is no history of injury then nearly all health concerns are related to bike set-up. It may be that you have noticed an obvious bike set-up error that may be the cause of the complaint, so you would ask the person to set the bike up as they usually would before a class. Advice on adjustments to positioning would be given at this stage.

If the complaint still causes discomfort please use Table 2.3.

Table 2.3	Health Concerns Solutions	
Complaint	Reason	Solution
Tiredness, lethargy, headaches	Dehydration/caffeinated drinks, stress	Drink at least one 500 ml bottle of water before/during and after the class
Saddle pain/irritation	Chafing from loose clothing	Wear fitted clothing/cycling shorts
	Saddle too high	Check bike set-up
	Sitting in middle of saddle	Vary position (back)
	Not supporting body with legs	Add more resistance
	Bobbing/bouncing in saddle	Press foot through bottom of shoe
		Use biomechanics
Male/female genital numbness	See above (bike set-up)	Change position in saddle
Toe numbness, pins and needles	Toe clips too tight	Loosen slightly
	Toes pushed to end of shoe	Vary foot position in shoe
	Footwear not offering support	Change footwear/buy proper bike shoes with rigid sole and/or cleats
Neck and shoulder pain/tension	Handlebars too low/high	Check bike set-up
	Too tense when cycling	Relax neck and drop shoulders/arms, loosen grip
Knee pain	Saddle too high/low	Check bike set-up;
	Fore and aft incorrect	Check natural 'gait' and adjust
	Unnatural knee position	foot position accordingly
Wrist pain, pins and needles	Pressure on wrists	Check bike set-up
	Not supporting body with legs	Roll knuckles over/out
		Add resistance
		Use biomechanics
Lower back ache	Normally lack of flexibility	Handlebars too low too soon
		Check bike set-up
		Poor biomechanics

VISUALISATION, FOCUS AND CONCENTRATION

These three words convey what are undoubtedly some of the most important aspects of studio cycling; the only limitation to which is the instructor and class's imagination. If you strengthen the mind the body will follow. If you have ever competed in a race you will know that you cannot win unless your body is trained to a superior level; however, in order to achieve that level you have to have a strong mind to achieve the training, proving the point that you cannot have one without the other.

This area of studio cycling can be misunderstood. The aim is to incorporate sports psychology principles and techniques into a studio environment and with a high heart rate. Properly used, it will enhance a person's training enormously, not just in the way they train but in the way they feel when training.

Coaching points:

- Start by closing your eyes and getting your clients to do the same; this blocks out visual distractions.
- Now imagine and explore with your senses; you may feel the wind in your face or smell freshly cut grass. Concentrating on such things helps you to lose consciousness of your actual surroundings.

Visualisation for example: *As you ride along you can see a long, straight, flat road. You can feel the heat of the sun on your back., the wind in your face. You can smell the freshly cut grass in the field next to the road, and hear the noises of your training partners' bikes and bodies as they cycle next to you.*

In this sentence we have used four senses to help visualisation. Different senses will be stronger in some people than others. You may even find that you cannot focus for long enough to concentrate on anything. Once you have achieved your image your goal is to keep yourself and your clients' heart rate elevated whilst spinning the pedals. If you are finding it tough try and visualise a road you know – everyone has a hill that they dread climbing or one they would love to climb. Perhaps you may have been watching the Tour de France and would like to take part, do whatever inspires you.

Your goal is to constantly try to reach this image. You will soon find that you are able to hold it for long periods of time and will be able to close your eyes and 'see' it. When you get to that stage try doing it with your eyes open; when this becomes easy it is time to find a new image. You have already started to develop a strong mind.

Everyone is different and you may even find that some of your clients will cheat. Remember to tell them that if any other thought comes into their heads the image is broken; even if they can return to it straightaway, they must be honest. To enhance this visualisation it must be done with a positive attitude, such as seeing ourselves with the perfect relaxed form. The power of the mind can tap potential that we thought was beyond ourselves!

Mental training

In order to practise or teach successful focus and visualisation techniques it is important to follow basic rules:

⚘ Start by closing eyes to cut out distractions.

⚘ Keep the visualisation familiar so people can relate to it (somewhere you know or have seen or been before).

⚘ Keep the visualisation positive (it's warm, you feel good, you are leading the race, you are achieving your goal).

⚘ Have a goal so people focus (we can see the top of the hill, the finish line is 200 metres away).

⚘ Give your visualisations an interval. For example, hold the image for one minute or one song.

⚘ Be progressive, lengthen the interval, change the challenges. You can incorporate progressive games in the form of challenges to hold an image as long as possible. Give the class some distractions like lack of music, or out-of-context commands. See who can stay focused the longest.

Senses

Also by using a variety of senses visualisation and concentration become more effective and realistic.

1 Sight – you can see the road ahead of you.

2 Feeling – you can feel the sun on your forearms and the breeze on your face.

3 Sound– you can hear the sound of the rider breathing next to you.

4 Smell – you can smell the freshly cut grass in the field next to you.

5 Taste – you can taste the energy drink in the water bottle.

6 Intuition – the sixth sense is used by most instructors without them even knowing it. The body language (visual feedback) that class members project to you will tell you vital information. Intuitively you will make decisions about the class (see feedbacks).

Relaxing

To relax is to enhance our power. In all great performance comes a form of physical, mental and emotional relaxation. If we can learn to relax when under stress then success is round the corner. As the workload gets harder and the heart rate increases so our bodies start to tense up; this is the time to teach yourself to listen to your body and relax! Use your breathing, visualisation and body-part list to help find **relaxation**. This will increase the blood flow and make the muscles more flexible.

Table 3.1	Focus Programme: example for class I
Warm-up	**Visualisation emphasis**: find a flat road; it's a beautiful day, feel the warm sun, hear your training partners riding next to you.
Pre-main set	Close your eyes and look down below your bike. See the white line and the road below the bike. As you go faster the gap between the white lines gets shorter.
Main set	Start a bike race with your friends, build in challenges of hills, flats, corners. See yourself in front – how does it feel? See yourself leading the race, pass a rider with a blue jersey on, pass with perfect strong technique, see yourself winning!
Recovery	Ride away from the finish to recover, away from the crowds, and find yourself all alone, strong, happy and relaxed.

Table 3.2	Focus Programme: example for class 2
Warm-up	**Music emphasis**: use music that inspires and says something to you, that makes you feel like riding in the mountains.
Pre-main set	**Technique emphasis**: focus on biomechanics, explore each muscle on both legs, hold each 'feel' for 20 seconds. Alternate the legs, count the strokes and change at each 50th stroke. Change the pace and count the cadence at each pace change. Hold for a count of 20.
Main set	**Music and breathing emphasis**: play an emotive piece of music to ride a flat road at a high tempo with a leg speed of 110 rpm. Use breathplay™ with intervals.
Recovery	**Music and visualisation emphasis**: pick a slower, more relaxing soundtrack that makes you proud of your efforts. See yourself on your way home feeling and looking great.
Post-class	Stretch off the bike and feel the muscles relax one by one, slow and lengthen the breathing pattern.

The Zone

By using all the progressive training elements including mental training you will have a chance to get into the 'Zone'. This is that euphoric state of mind when everything seems easy. You feel you could ride forever at that pace. These are the rides that keep you coming back. However, one thing you must realise is that it is easy to over train in rides like this. Human nature and the human mind can play tricks, and sometimes you can do one session too many.

Coaching and mental training

The way we learn is important to understand and in the book *Body Language and Mentality* by Anthony Robins we can learn how different people pick up information from our method of coaching. See if you can recognise yourself as a visual, auditory or kinaesthetic learner, or, probably, a mixture of all three.

Coaching and communication

A coach is someone who can influence and guide an individual. With their knowledge, experience, empathy and guidance they can put a person on an individual studio-cycling training programme even within the group, and give them completely different techniques and challenges than the rest of the class if required, allowing them to work at their own level and pace. A coach is professional and has the ability to communicate to the person exactly when and what they need to do to progress. A coach has the skill to help the client set goals and work through the training process to achieve and then reset them.

A coach is only as good as the delivery of what she or he is trying to say and do; for instance, through their choice of words, voice tonality and body language they can convey exactly what it is they need the person to know. This is a skill and will be learnt and developed over time. Everyone is an individual and the coach will learn, too, from every new client worked with.

Table 3.3	Visual, auditory and kinaesthetic types of people		
	Visual type	**Auditory type**	**Kinaesthetic type**
Language	Talks in pictures	Well-aimed choice of words	Slower reactions, sensitive
Voice	Talks fast, high voice	Sonorous, with rhythm	Deep voice
Linguistic ability	Superficial language. A person that is thinking faster than he/she is speaking. Oversupply of pictures and lack of competence to find the correct words	Slow talker. Well-pointed words	Quiet most of the time, sensitive formulations
Phrasing	Describes pictures, uses words connected with sight: "I can see that you are doing well." "I can imagine it."	Uses words connected with hearing: "That sounds good."	Very often uses material pictures, concrete descriptions; needs to get a feeling for the subject
Breathing	Very high in the lungs, flat	Uses lunges and diaphragmatic breathing	Diaphragmatic breathing
Position of the head	Keeps head high	Keeps head high or lowered	Head lowered

If you do not maintain eye contact when conveying a technique to the class you can be perceived as lacking in confidence and being uncertain. Look people in the eyes! Keep your head up, be expressive with your body language. A smile or nod at the right time is worth a hundred words!

> 55% of communication comes from body language.
> 38% of communication comes from voice tonality.
> 7% of communication comes from the actual words we say.
>
> *Impact of Presentation (Joseph O'Conner, John Seymour 1994)*

If you talk quietly you can be perceived as having low self esteem, and speaking indistinctly will give the impression that you teach carelessly. Change the tone, rhythm, depth, speed and range of your voice. Be clear, audible and positive and assume control of the class.

Receiving feedback

There are three types of feedback that a studio-cycling instructor should look for and constantly be aware of before, during and after a class.

1 Instructor's/coach's visual observation
Look for signs in your class of how people

feel. Face and body movements will be sending you signals about how they are responding and whether they are coping with your class. As you get to know the individuals you will start to gauge how they are progressing or if there are underlying problems. As a studio instructor your job isn't just to teach a class – you are a coach, a third eye and a friend. For some people, you will be the only one they can talk to. They will respect your opinions and look to you for guidance. Don't let them down, have patience with them and give thoughtful advice. Be sensitive if you recognise negative signals, perhaps wait till the end of the class before you ask someone how they're doing – it may be something personal and too private a matter to discuss in front of the class.

Quite often someone will be overstressed and a simple comment will make them realise there is a problem and they can make adjustments. That person will not forget your help!

If a regular member doesn't seem to respond as normal, or perhaps looks different (maybe you can't quite put your finger on it), don't dismiss your perception of that person; trust your instinct and intuition that something may be wrong. A simple, general comment to the whole class may address the situation, such as, 'Everybody relax! This class is for you, forget the things outside the class', then look that person in the eye. They may make the necessary change, or you may perhaps make a mental note to talk to that person after the class. They will respect you for your concern, professionalism and help.

2 Verbal observation – rate of perceived exertion (RPE)

Until the use of heart rate monitoring, RPE was primarily used to help gauge the level of intensity at which someone thought they were working. A coach would communicate the intensity required with RPE as to what level they were to work at and to what level they thought they were working. This is still an important area as many people don't have a heart rate monitor (which is more accurate, except the heart rate can play tricks on you).

RPE has played an important part in the role of a coach over the years. It is simple to use and can help you explain your requirements to a class or individual as well as assisting with goal setting. Use a scale of 1–10:

1 is asleep (easy), 10 is as hard as you can ever go (maximum).

Practical guidelines to use in your class are:

Warm-up	5<7
Main class	7<9
Warm-down	7>5
Finish	5>3

Before the start clients should be at 3–4 (more than this indicates that the student may be overtrained, tired, or negatively stressed).

With experience your warm-down will help clients to de-stress and recover. Quite often after a well-structured class clients will feel euphoric.

3 Observing people

It is a vital part of being an instructor that you analyse the following:

- What will make people come in the first place?
- Why should they come again, and what will it take to create a successful studio-cycling programme for each individual?

In time, an instructor will get to know who each person is, why they are in the class, what they have done before, and what will make them come again and again.

To start with, we can break down into four types the people who will make up the class, so that it becomes a challenge to teach and coach.

TYPE 1: Mr/Mrs Stressed

He or she will probably have just rushed from work and is generally stressed. You will use your skills of visualisation and the added stress-reducing benefits of exercise to make them feel better. They may need a longer warm-up and pre-main set than others in your class.

TYPE 2: Mr/Mrs Ballistic

He or she will have lots of energy and want to go hard from the start. They often don't want to listen to your guidance of RPE, they are usually quite fit but probably overtrained and one step away from injury. Sometimes it's best to let them go off hard at the start and soon enough as you ask the group to work harder they will be working so hard they have to slow down and will then listen to your commands. Generally this sort of person will always want to work near their maximum.

TYPE 3: Mr/Mrs Journey

This student wants to be led on a journey and forget everything else. The instructor will have the skill to let him or her forget what they are doing and train them while they are thinking about something else, making the time fly by and them feel great. They are very receptive to information and take what you say seriously so it is imperative that you give them the right instruction and commands to stop them learning bad habits. Don't do anything stupid as they are likely to follow. You can tell the real journey people when you scratch your head – a few in the class will do the same because they think it's part of the training.

TYPE 4: Mr/Mrs Focused

This client needs to stimulate the mind and take themselves out of the studio to another place. They can leave the studio and be somewhere where they want to be by using their imagination and the triggers from the instructor, strengthening concentration and building focus through strong visualisation techniques. You will

not have to speak as much to them as they have been taught the correct skills from the start and are working in their zone.

> **Instructor tip:**
>
> Our goal is for a stressed or ballistic person to become a journey person. Then we want the journey people to become the focused people. The person with the strong mind will ultimately reach her or his goals.

Coaching and motivation

The skill to motivate individuals comes naturally to some but to others it can be developed and learnt.

In this section, identify what motivations you have used before, or what you feel comfortable with using or want to try. To keep people coming regularly to your classes – indeed, to get them to come in the first place – is a real skill; learn it and your classes will always be full.

There are two kinds of motivation; secondary, which is external and can be because of the coach, or primary, internal motivation, where the goal itself can be the motivating factor. Secondary motivation could be stressful if, for instance, someone is doing a class just because they have been told to. However if you can turn someone to have primary motivation, i.e. they want to join the class in order to reach the goal, they are more likely to be consistent. We can achieve this by setting different goals.

Goal-setting

Goals are achievable dreams! The way to reach those goals is to set yourself realistic targets. They are time-linked, which means that a time must be set to complete them, which is why we have short-, medium- and long-term goals.

Short-term goals (STG): these can be class or daily goals. Within a class uses sets and challenges.

- Use the principles of frequency, intensity, time and type (FITT).
- The challenge – set the challenge for the class based on current fitness levels, how they are responding to their effort, what previous training they have done, i.e. if they have been doing intervals, then see how you can progress them. For example:

1 A seated flat interval of 6×1 minute efforts at 80% cadence 90 rpm could progress to 8×1 minute at 80% cadence 90 rpm. The goal is to add two more intervals therefore progressing the frequency.

2 6×1 minute efforts at 80% could progress to 6×1 minute efforts at 85%. The goal is to increase intensity from 80% to 85%. The intensity can be added by adding resistance and watching the heart rate percent, or increasing the rpm (remember the cadence guidelines for the set terrain).

3 6×1 minute efforts at 80% could progress to 4×2 minutes or 6×80 seconds at 80%. The goal is to add extra time, which can be either reducing the intervals but lengthening the time of each one, or adding time to each interval and maintaining the number.

4 Seated flat interval of 6×1 minute at 80%, change the technique to standing flat. Keep the heart rate percent the same. Obviously the technique can change in many ways with all the other techniques available. The goal is to maintain the heart rate but change the technique.

Medium-term goals (MTG): these could be setting up a training programme or measuring heart rate responses such as resting heart rate, delta heart rate and recovery heart rate. These can show improvement within weeks. See heart zones tests.

Long-term goals (LTG): these could be fat loss, race results, completing an endurance event. A goal could be set over months or even years (see Goal Setting chart).

Technique

Techniques set at the correct time will motivate the class; for example, 'climb a mountain to an extreme height'. There will be other factors such as choice of music, the correct tempo and timing, how long the technique lasts and, if the motivation or enthusiasm seems low, the skill to change the technique and remotivate the class; these must be put together with a blend of progression and skill. Emphasise technique skills such as biomechanics and muscle stability and measure improvements.

Praise and encouragement

Use key words to motivate your clients by giving them praise and encouragement, such as 'Well done!', 'You're looking great', 'Feel strong', 'See yourself winning, ahead of the pack', 'Fantastic', 'Focus on yourself', 'Be one with the bike', 'You're a winner!' etc, etc. They must be positive and encouraging.

Eye contact

Sometimes eye contact will be all that is needed to motivate someone to work harder or correct their technique, re-focus and concentrate. It can be a very powerful and external communicator that gives you an option away from an autocratic style. You will know the style best suited to your personality. Use what works for you but keep an open mind and maybe work on your weakness to build confidence and a larger skills base.

Example of a Goal Setting chart					
Students should tick which of these reasons and aims for participating in exercise applies to them:					
Goals	Tick	Goal type (STG, MTG or LTG)	Goals	Tick	Goal type (STG, MTG or LTG)
1. Improved fitness/healthier lifestyle			2. Competitive sport		
3. Doctor's advice			4. Health improvements		
5. To tone and improve body shape			6. Stress reduction		
7. Weight loss			8. Social reasons		

Body language

Along with eye contact goes mimicry. If you see poor technique you can search for eye contact with the person. Once they are looking at you, emphasise perfect technique, and show them what you are looking for with your body language. If they don't pick up on this, copy their poor technique then show them how to correct it. All this can be done without saying anything and is a stronger style than picking on someone who may be embarrassed.

Teamwork

Riding the techniques together with synergy is a fantastic way to achieve a quick response and motivate the group. There are many different games you can play:

- Follow the leader: the instructor leads a technique and the class follows, or pick a strong rider to be leader.
- Team teach: two to four instructors face the class and lead techniques one at a time. This will build strong, respected teams of leaders.

Each instructor can be introduced by the preceding one.

- Mimicry games: class members copy everything the instructor does without anyone talking. The techniques can last for 30 seconds or 5 minutes depending on the programme.
- Studio-cycling wars: the instructor starts a technique and everyone has to follow changes in techniques and gear changes (resistance). This can be done with one leader or in pairs, swapping from one leader to another. Another option is to get the pairs to fight with techniques. This means one person leads, and as soon as the other person is bored they can change the lead with a new technique; this can swap constantly or within a set period of time.
- Leg speeds: the instructor sets leg-speed guidelines and the class will ride at that speed. As the rpms change the class has to match. The instructor can teach the class how to count cadence. Each time the leg touches the elbow on one side counts as one revolution. Count for 6 seconds and add a

nought. Increasing and decreasing the numbers with equal resistance can be used for warm-ups, challenges and recoveries.

- Techniques in unison: everyone has to stay together for certain techniques such as combination flats or hills or standing climb. The legs all spin in the same time with one leg on the same side leading. Alternate the lead leg when the group gets tired, or build into the programme the balance if one leg is slower or weaker than the other one.
- Sports-specific techniques or games (see *Studio Cycling for Teams* and *Athletes Spin to Win*).

Motivation is such an important part of exercise, not just in terms of studio cycling but in the whole of life: without motivation you will not even get out of bed! Perhaps that is why people set goals whether they be short-, medium- or long-term goals, each one is specific to the individual and an excellent motivator. In studio-cycling terms, motivation is vital and is what makes people return to the same class again and again. Instructors need to be aware of the teaching tips of motivation; as we mentioned, eye contact, praise and encouragement are all powerful forms of communication. However, if you as an instructor feel that verbal motivation works best for you and your clients, you are the one best placed to decide. Teamwork is an excellent way to motivate the class and the instructor; whether it takes the form of challenging class member against class member or of 'team teaching' both methods are equally rewarding. Motivation is the key to making your classes a success both for yourself and for your members.

| Fig. 3.1 | Studio-cycling class using film footage |

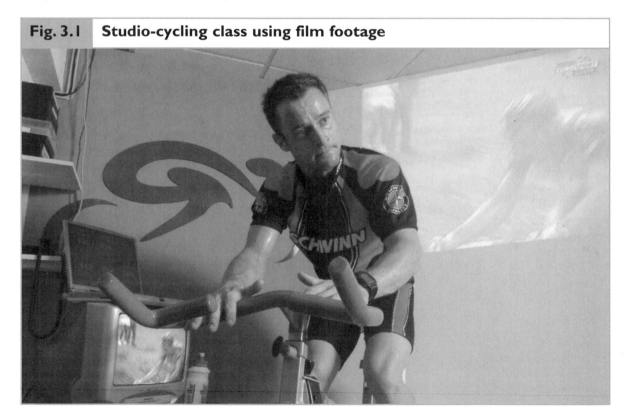

What of the future?

Recently we have seen the introduction of 'super' external motivators in the form of projection screens showing amazing scenes of cycling footage. We can watch the Tour de France Stage Races in the Alps; the packs on the road; the effort on the faces; the sheer beauty of the scenery; and the machines as they climb effortlessly! These really can inspire people as long as they are played at the right time. We have found that in order to follow a mind/body work-out it is best to train these areas first before you put on these pictures. We want to train people with strong minds who can focus without needing an image. However, such film footage can create an amazing experience for some, and the look on their faces when Lance Armstrong comes on the screen, hammering up Alp Duez is wonderful!!

However, it should be kept for advanced classes as otherwise individuals might get super-motivated and work too hard too soon.

There are now also computer software and scanners that can put the heart rates of large groups of people up on the screen (see Fig. 3.2). It is important that class members do not rely on these for motivation, but you can use them to get that extra 5% out of the class if necessary. However, unless you know what the numbers for your class mean, they will be useless. The next chapter will teach you how to use heart rate monitoring as a motivating tool.

Fig. 3.2   Studio-cycling class with heart rate display

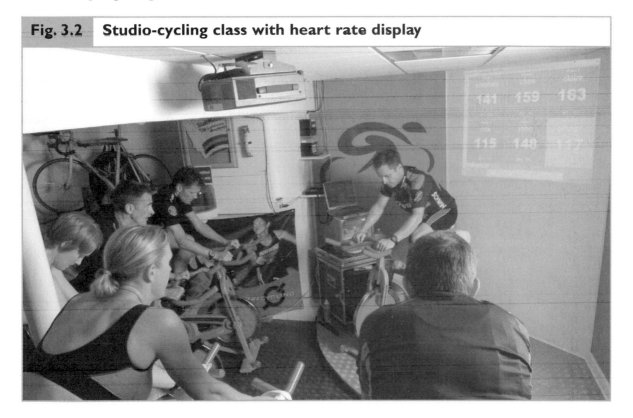

HEART ZONE TRAINING FOR STUDIO CYCLING

Why use a heart rate monitor?

Of all the feedbacks available for studio cycling, heart rate monitoring has to be the most accurate! The other feedbacks such as visual and verbal can be great communicators and are vital for class success, but for accuracy and motivation there is no better and user-friendly response or feedback than the heart response.

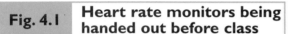

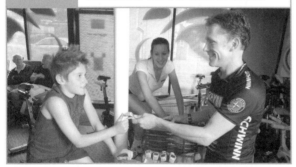

Fig. 4.1 — **Heart rate monitors being handed out before class**

The heart is a muscle that pumps all the time; even in the most sedentary of people. If the heart does not function we cease to live. When the body is exerted and the heart responds by pumping faster to cope with the extra workload it needs to adapt very quickly, especially as there might be more exertion later (the mind thinks it knows everything!), so in response it grows and gets stronger very quickly. This fact is extremely useful for motivation within a training programme, and measuring and monitoring the heart from the beginning will increase the likelihood of an individual sticking consistently to the programme. An instructor should start to talk about the heart rate before,

during and after the class. Take the heart rate manually; as the clients learn about the heart and their own personal responses they will want a monitor on their wrist so they can see it all the time. Sell the concept of heart rate monitoring in Zone 2, (60–70%). (See Fig. 4.3.)

What is a heart rate monitor?

If your programme is to be a success, to get the most accuracy you will need the help of a cheap and simple tool. Heart Zone Training™ is the software and the heart rate monitor is the tool or the computer. A heart monitor will provide biofeedback about the heart. It will accurately display the average number of times the heart contracts in one minute by picking up the electrical signals given off by the heart. Heart rate monitors today use a transmitter (chest strap and belt) worn against the skin underneath the chest. In some cases where this is uncomfortable the bulky part of the belt can be worn round the middle of the back. Normally this needs to be dampened to enable a strong signal to go to the receiver. The transmitter receives data from the heart through its electrodes, processes the signals then sends it to the receiver (monitor). Sometimes if an unusual number is seen, often at the start of the work-out, it is the transmitter trying to locate all the many signals of electricity it is receiving. After a few minutes it starts to recognise the true heart rate and becomes accurate.

The receiver (monitor) is in the form of a watch that can be fastened around the wrist or in some cases mounted on the handlebars. It is the receiver that carries most of the interesting and useful functions. However, the most important numbers will be the displayed heart rate in beats per minute (bpm). Normally the more functions a heart monitor has the more expensive it is. It is hoped that the next generation of heart monitors will not need the belt and strap as they can become sweaty and need regular cleaning.

Fig. 4.2 **Heart monitor being attached**

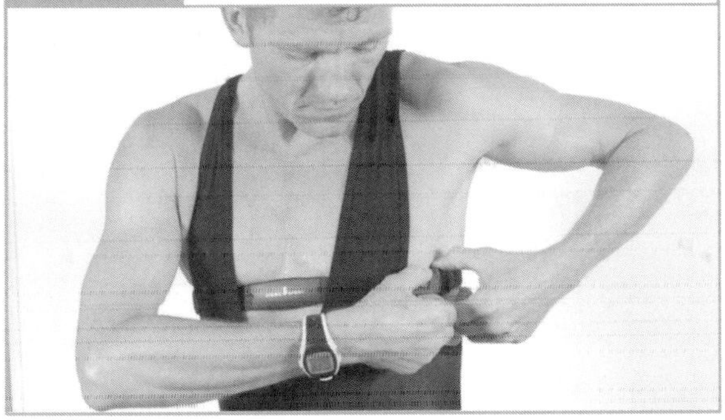

How to use a heart rate monitor

Sometimes the best way to introduce a new concept is simply to 'just do it!' and this can be the same way with the heart rate monitor. Just put it on and see what happens in a work-out. Clubs can now purchase 'station bags' that carry 10–15 heart monitors that can be handed out to clients to try before they buy their own. The instructor should ask the client to look at the numbers, to measure the heart rate before the work-out (ambient heart rate) and during the different intensities (peaks); remember also to measure it at recovery. How long does the heart rate take to come down after a specific effort or intensity? Already the client or athlete is learning about the body and its responses. This feedback will become invaluable later on in the programme, both to measure improvement and to motivate the individual. This can be a quick learning process and the

education will continue as the zone numbers are discovered, a dosage of time in zones prescribed and the programme followed.

In the past instructors and coaches have used the maximum heart rate as an anchor point from which to determine the percentages of heart rate an individual should work at. This great and simple idea has unfortunately long proved to be inaccurate. The formula '220 – age' was discovered in 1938 and picked up years later by the fitness industry. Heart monitor companies used it because it was simple; they built their products around it, because it allowed their customers to buy a monitor and start using it after a few simple calculations. However, it doesn't work for most of the population and due to this inaccuracy it has caused many people to discard their monitor and go back to the Rate of Perceived Exertion (RPE) scale, or, as most people do, 'just train!' There must be hundreds of thousands of heart monitors in cupboards and drawers or festering at the bottom of a damp kitbag.

Until recently this wasn't the only reason people didn't use heart monitors, another factor was their expense. The first monitors in the early 1980s were hundreds of dollars or pounds and many people couldn't justify the cost; there were not enough good reasons to have one. When people did buy one they found that the numbers were incorrect and didn't make sense. It can be very demotivating if the numbers say one thing and the formula says you should be at another level. Hence the market is still very untapped and you can still see even top athletes training without a monitor.

Sally Edwards, one of the world's leading authorities on heart rate training with a heart rate monitor, has developed a programme called Heart Zones® which is probably the most useful and user-friendly programme available. It can be incorporated in every studio-cycling class to great effect.

Fig. 4.3 Heart zone training chart

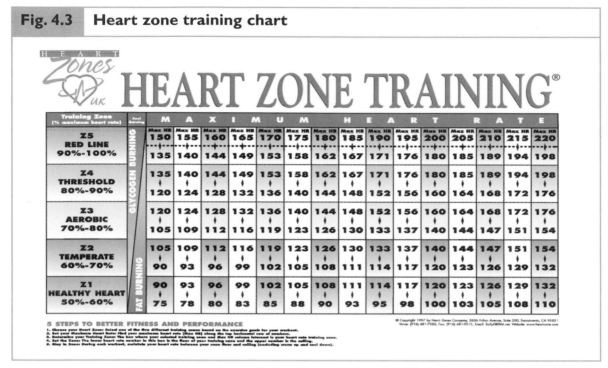

The Heart Zone Training® application uses a more accurate maximum heart rate as an anchor point to find five zones.

Characteristics of maximum heart rate

You may find these characteristics interesting and helpful in understanding why we use the maximum heart rate as our anchor point:

Fig. 4.4	Zone benefits
Blue Zone	Known as the Healthy Heart Zone – easiest and most comfortable zone. Benefits: Lowered blood pressure, lowered cholesterol, decreased risk of degenerative diseases
Green Zone	The Temperate Zone or Recovery Zone. Benefits: Healthy heart, fat mobilisation by moving fat from cell, fat to muscle, increase of mitochondria, increase of fat release from fat cell
Yellow Zone	Aerobic Zone or Transition Zone – shifting ratio of fuel. Benefits: Improved functional capacity, increase in number and size of blood vessels, respiratory rate, max pulmonary ventilation, pulmonary diffusion, increase in difference in arterial-venous oxygen, increase in size and strength of heart
Orange Zone	Threshold Zone – improved VO2 threshold and higher lactate tolerance ability
Red Zone	Red Zone – for performance and athletes. High interval zone. Also known as injury zone

- Your maximum heart rate (MHR) is the anchor point which Heart Zone Training® uses to find the five training zones.
- Your MHR is genetically determined: you are born with it, just like the colour of your eyes.
- Your MHR does *not* deteriorate with age.
- Your MHR is a fixed number, unless you become unfit.
- MHR can be affected by some medications.
- Your MHR, whether high or low, does not predict performance.
- MHR has great variability of people of the same age.
- Your MHR is sports specific; it will change depending on the sport, e.g. a runner could have a different MHR from a cyclist.

Characteristics of the zones

- All zones have a weight starting at 50–60%. The higher the zone the heavier the weight.
- All zones have a size of 10%.
- All zones have a floor, midpoint and ceiling.
- You cannot get the benefits of training in a low zone by training in a higher zone.
- All zones have multiple benefits – physiological changes, fuel consumption, individual feelings, time spent in zone and training effects.
- All zones form part of a progressive programme from health through fitness to performance.
- All zones are relative, which means that they are specific to the individual's maximum heart rate.

Useful heart numbers

As a way of measuring and monitoring progress we can use some very useful numbers: ambient heart rate, resting heart rate, delta heart rate and recovery heart rate.

Ambient heart rate

Ambient heart rate is measured when the body is awake but inactive. Some people confuse resting heart rate with ambient heart rate. Ambient heart rate will change depending on the external stimuli influences such as temperature, hydration, food ingestion, and internal influences such as fatigue, stress, hunger, sleep, insomnia and medication plus many others. Ambient heart rates are relative not absolute, and will need to be taken repeatedly for accurate assessment. The normal range of an ambient heart rate could be 50–90 bpm but a healthy range can be very wide. A high ambient heart rate will be relative to the above stresses mentioned but will reduce as you become fitter. An instructor should look for abnormally high ambient heart rates to make rest, recovery and frequency, intensity, time and type decisions for programme changes.

Resting heart rate

Resting heart rate is a great indicator of fitness, overtraining and stress as it measures parasympathetic nervous response. It should be taken in the morning a few minutes after you wake. When you wake your heart will soar as you move, stretch, open your eyes and take in the light and surroundings. Wait and it will drop again to where it was when you were at full rest or asleep. Take it manually for a full minute and record it, or put on your heart monitor and relax for a while to register a low for that morning.

With positive training effects resting heart rate can decrease, as the heart gets stronger and pumps more blood in one stroke, therefore contracting fewer times. This translates to less physiological stress. In terms of overall lifestyle this will result in as many as 700 million beats less over a lifetime for an individual with a lowered resting heart rate. Surely that is worth saving! Your resting heart rate will change from day to day depending on lifestyle. Are you sleeping poorly, overtraining, getting sick or stressed? These conditions affect resting heart rate by an increase of 5–10 beats or more! If abnormal changes occur due to training then the training programme can be adapted to allow the body to recover. The heart can be so responsive that I have seen my resting heart rate rise before I have been aware of the symptoms of illness. There are many benefits from a test that only takes one minute!

Delta heart rate

The delta heart rate, also known as orthostatic heart rate, is the heart's response to body position change. Delta (Δ) is a letter in the Greek alphabet conveying 'change'.

The test can be performed in an initial sitting or lying position and the heart rate recorded after 2 minutes. After this the individual should stand for 2 minutes and take a recording. The difference between the two indicates physical stress levels, which can be ideal to incorporate within a training programme. For instance after multiple readings, a change in results following exercise can help determine recovery time and intensity levels during subsequent training. The test should be conducted prior to workload, for example at the same time each morning before breakfast.

Individuals who exercise regularly should use the prone or lying to standing positions.

To find your delta heart rate:

Lie down for 2 minutes; your heart rate will drop to be close to that of your resting heart rate (see Fig 4.5)

Now stand. The cardiac system adjusts to this change in body position. It will first increase, then drop to a new value after 2 minutes. The difference between these two figures is the delta heart rate.

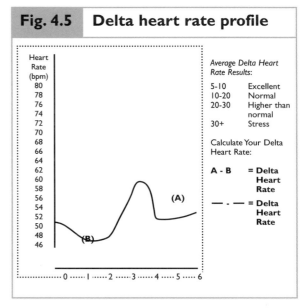

Fig. 4.5 Delta heart rate profile

You can use the scale in the box to interpret the results (see Fig. 4.6).

Fig. 4.6 Delta Results

0–10 bpm: Normal. You can continue with the training programme.

11–20 bpm: Caution. Keep an eye on how you feel and monitor any changes or responses.

21–30 bpm: Be aware. This could show high amounts of stress, a compromised immune system, medications. You should train in a lower zone.

30+ bpm: Take action. Either you are overtraining and need to take a day off or you have another response that requires action and could require retesting until you see a drop below 30 bpm. If the rate continues to he high and you have been following a cardiovascular training programme for a while you might feel reassured after a visit to the doctor.

The delta heart rate assessment should be taken over a few days and any variation observed. Once a normal delta heart rate has been established it can then be taken after high intensity work-outs. If there are significant changes the individuals and coaches can look back at the programme and identify and rectify the cause. Normally rest and recovery is sufficient. This will fit into a pattern that can be seen from your training diary.

Recovery heart rate

Recovery heart rate can be measured after a certain predetermined heart rate is reached. The recovery heart rate will be the number of beats measured over a time period of normally 1–2 minutes. The higher the drop the stronger the heart is becoming. This measurement can become very useful as a tool to motivate an individual (see Chapter 3). The instructor or coach can build these tests into existing work-outs or classes.

Example 1: recovery test protocol
Mary, a 39-year-old accountant, follows a training programme written by her personal trainer. She has been training for 3 months from a base of very little and inconsistent training in the past. Her goal is to get fit, lose fat weight and tone up, although she doesn't need to lose too much. She would like to take part in the London to Brighton charity bike ride next year. Her coach gave her a fitness test at the start of her programme including fat percentage, lung function, blood pressure, flexibility and several sub-maximal tests on a stationary bike to predict her maximum heart rate for cycling. It was predicted to be 200 bpm. From this she can quickly work out her heart zones which are as follows:

100% = 200 bpm	80% = 160 bpm	60% = 120 bpm
90% = 180 bpm	70% = 140 bpm	50% = 100 bpm

The day before her recovery test work-out she has a rest day. Today's work-out is on a road bike outside. Mary will ride for 1 hour.

Warm-up: She follows the usual 10-minute warm up – Zone 1–2 (50% <60%).

Pre-main set: Zone 2 progressive intervals to elevate her heart rate to the ceiling of Zone 2 (60%<70%) for 5 minutes.

Main Set: Once ready her coach has asked her to ride at the ceiling of Zone 2 for 10 minutes (70%), increase to midpoint of Zone 3 over the next 5 minutes (75%). She will hold this pace for 5 minutes then build the heart rate up to the ceiling of Zone 3 (up to 80%) and hold for the next 15 minutes.

Recovery: At this points she stops and measures her recovery over 1 minute. After this she continues to warm-down through the zones for 9 minutes.

Results: Mary held 160 bpm (80%) for 15 minutes then measured recovery for 1 minute, her heart rate dropped to 136 bpm giving a recovery rate of 24 bpm. This is logged in her training diary and will be repeated in 4 weeks' time after following a structured and progressive programme. The higher the recovery number the fitter she becomes and the nearer her goal she gets.

Conclusions: By taking a recovery heart rate Mary and her coach can see very quickly if the training is working. Repeating the tests periodically and looking for small or significant changes is the key to making these tests work for you.

You can make up your own tests but stick rigidly to the same protocol each time and try to repeat the same test conditions, such as a recovery period before the test, same time of day, same temperature, same equipment (stationary bike), plenty of hydration and foods. Then you will have an accurate test and the results will be valid. Improvements can be seen almost straight away.

Table 4.1	Results of exercise in different zones				
Zone heart rate	% of max. burnt	Fuels burnt for 30 mins	Calories	RPE of feeling	Description
5	90–100% 10% fat 1% protein	90% carb	450–600	9–10	Very tough, extremely strenuous
4	80–90% 15% fat 1% protein	85% carb	<420	7–8	Very tough to hard
3	70–80% 45% fat 5% protein	50% carb	<330	5–6	Strong to heavy
2	60–70% 70% fat 5% protein	25% carb	<240	3–4	Moderate to strong
1	50–60% 85% fat 5% protein	10% carb	<180	1–2	Light to easy

Using a heart monitor for weight management

Many people ask questions regarding fat and weight loss related to studio-cycling training. The questions below are some of the most frequently asked; in reading the answers it is important to remember that everyone is different – we all display highly individual differences in response to food as fuel.

In what zone can I burn the most fat?

The answer is not as simple as dedicating fat utilisation to one zone; it very much depends on your level of fitness. The fitter you are the more fat can be burned in each zone, for example an unfit person would burn the most fat in the lower range, from 2 to 3. If you are extremely fit, you will burn the most fat in Zone 4 or 5. However, for long-term weight management, the important point is the number of calories you burn rather than the percentage of fat. In order to burn fat, oxygen must be present. If you exercise aerobically with plenty of oxygen without shortness of breath, you burn a high percentage of fat. As soon as you cross over to the anaerobic exercise intensity, the point where there is not enough oxygen to sustain the exercise, you don't burn any additional fat.

What fuel types are burnt in each zone?

A different ratio of fuel is burnt in each of the five heart zones. The higher the heart rate or the level of exercise intensity the higher the percentage of fat calories used. If your goals are long-term weight management research suggests that burning a higher number of calories can help, therefore the best solution is to spend longer periods of time in zones that you can sustain (see Table 4.1).

Does everyone burn calories differently?

Absolutely. A calorie is not simply a measurement of the way we burn or metabolise energy. Energy balance is completely individual. There are many different factors in achieving an energy shift that can result in successful weight management.

1 The ratio of fuels in your current diet: if you eat a high fat diet you'll burn a higher percentage of fat when you train.
2 Your current fitness level: the fitter you are, the more fat you'll burn at the same exercise intensity.
3 What you have just eaten.

So how do I expand my fat burning range?

Most people make the mistake of thinking that to burn most fat you have to train in the lower zones. In reality you would have to train for hours daily for months to make significant and noticeable fat reductions. You have two thresholds, T1 and T2. T1 (approx. 50–55%) is where you start to burn fat and T2 (approx. 85–90%) is where you stop burning extra fat. The key is to raise T2 so that you burn fat over a greater range. To do this you must train in all the zones and build in proactive rest. You cannot change your maximum heart rate but you can change your threshold T2. Endurance athletes will race at their best when they have a high threshold.

How to find predicted maximum heart rate, before or during the class, and anaerobic threshold

There are different tests we can perform to find an accurate maximum heart rate without carrying out an actual 'maximum test', which is not very user-friendly. It hurts, and can only be done with someone who is healthy, has an exercise background and has signed a waiver stating that they understand the test protocol and agree that it is at their own risk. In the US fire service up to 25 years ago more firemen were killed doing their fitness tests than in fires, because of the extreme severity of maximal and VO_2 tests. We need to use simple and accurate sub-max tests that can be administered simply before a class, individually, or during a class, as a group. These tests can be structured in by a skilled instructor so that the class doesn't even know they are doing them until afterwards. However, you may find it better to outline them to the class so that they know what is expected of them beforehand and can be prepared.

There are 6–10 different sub-max tests that can be performed by most of your class members. However, some tests are easier than others and it is important for you to know which test will suit which fitness level of riders. We have included a selection for you to use. Some can be carried out within your normal class timetable. If you wish to find out more about the other tests contact Heart Zones UK (see reference at end of book).

You must also familiarise yourself with Rate of Perceived Exertion (RPE) Scale, as we have previously discussed. You can choose which scale you prefer as long as you use it consistently.

The tests:

A Studio- cycling sub-max test
B The 'Every Two Minutes Go Harder' test
C Cycling anaerobic threshold test
D Studio-cycling fitness test
E Core temperature starts to heat up but in control
F If you have ever used a heart rate monitor and you have perceived yourself to work hard, what is the highest number you have seen.

Studio-cycling sub-max test

Try this test that uses your Perceived Rate of Exertion (RPE) i.e. how you feel, with an

Table 4.2	Protocol chart		
RPE scale	Add bpm	Feeling	% of max HR
1	90	Very little effort	
2	80	Easy	Less than 35%
3	70	Moderate	35–50%
4	60	Somewhat strong	50–60%
5	50	Strong but comfortable	60–70%
6	40	Challenging	70–80%
7	30	Very strong	80–85%
8	20	Hard/deep breathing	85–90%
9	10	Very very hard	90–95%
10	0	Ready to stop	95–100%

Results Table			
RPE	Heart rate	Add bpm	Predicted max HR
	110bpm	+	=
	120 bpm	+	=
	130 bpm	+	=
	140 bpm	+	=
	150 bpm	+	=
	160 bpm	+	=
	170 bpm	+	=
	180 bpm	+	=
	190 bpm	+	=
		Average total	=

intensity level combined with your current fitness and the numbers on your heart rate monitor.

Protocol:

- Warm up for 5–10 minutes at about 90–100 bpm
- Increase heart rate to 110 bpm and maintain for 2 minutes, then record the RPE number and increase heart rate to 120 bpm. At the end of the following 2 minutes record the RPE number and increase the heart rate to 130 bpm. Repeat the sequence increasing the heart rate by 10 beats.
- The test stops when the RPE number is 7 or higher, if lower than 7 continue to elevate the heart rate in 10-beat increments.
- Recover for 5 minutes or until heart rate is measured below 100 bpm.

The 'every two minutes go harder' test

This test will use your subjective feeling of exercise intensity or RPE in a scale of 1–10. We have simplified this scale so that it is easy to use for everyone. After you have warmed up you will spend 2 minutes at each number in the scale until you feel challenged or tired.

Scale: 1 = Asleep
3 = Walking around
4 = Light effort
5 = Easy and heating up
6 = Steady state
7 = Involved
8 = Hard – but sustainable
8.5 = Very hard (this is approximately most people's threshold, where they cross from aerobic to anaerobic, with and without oxygen)
9 = Very, very hard
10 = Maximum – as hard as you can go

Start – warm up for 5–10 minutes. Go at an easy pace, ensure you are feeling comfortable. After around 5 minutes you should start to feel warm, after 10 minutes or less you will be feeling hot and maybe starting to perspire.

At this point you may start. For 2 minutes, ride at each number as described in the RPE scale. If you are starting out on a training programme you should only ride to a 7 on the RPE scale. However, you can repeat this test and ride the numbers as many times as you like to compare the data. All tests like these are relative to your lifestyle and whatever is affecting you at present, such as stress, lack of sleep, illness etc. At a 7 you will be at approximately 70% (see the Heart Zones Chart, Fig. 4.3)

Cycling anaerobic threshold test

This test can be done within a tough 2 × 20 minutes workout. This test is a very accurate way of determining your anaerobic threshold, which, remember, changes every day. Think about the times when training was easy, you could get your heart rate high and you seemed to float through the work-out or race. That was when your threshold was high. It was then that you burnt the most fat! On another day you might have felt lethargic and sluggish, you struggled to raise your heart rate without going extremely hard. That was when your threshold was low. Now think about both – what was the difference? Start by looking at lifestyle: had you slept badly, trained and not recovered? Were you stressed, or suffering with a cold? These things will lower your threshold. On a day like that, don't push it, don't race! Take a day off!

Here is a test that will enable you to find your threshold:
Protocol:
- Cycle as hard as you can for 20 minutes.
- Follow with a 5-minute recovery.
- Again, cycle as hard as you can 20 minutes.
- Recover.

If you cycled as hard as you could you have an excellent indicator of your current anaerobic threshold. The test should be done after a period of a day or more, conditions should be constant each time do it. The client must do this test after a rest. The higher the threshold the more fat you burn; tests have shown this is the upper heart rate of the fat-burning range. You will become fitter and faster.

A test such as this is ideal for setting heart rate race pace in endurance competitions, although remember it is sports-specific and test-day sensitive so you must repeat the test a few times and change sport if you wish to find the most accurate anaerobic threshold for your actual sport.

Studio-cycling fitness test

This test can be fun and a little competitive between the class members, but healthy because everyone is always working at their own level. It can be modified to suit the present fitness level of class members and adapted as they progress. It will be a challenging and exhilarating work-out.

After the warm-up and pre-main set where the heart rate has been elevated to 75% of max the test can begin. The duration is 10 minutes and controlled by the class members themselves. The instructor will provide motivating music, time checks and the rules, which are: over 10 minutes, see how many times you can elevate your heart rate to 85% then drop it immediately to 65%; repeat this as many times as possible in the period. See Figure 4.7 for how the profile can look for a fit person. It doesn't matter how many 'spikes' there are; the key is to train, get fitter and add more spikes as you improve. The usual test will see a drop of around 40 bpm but beginner classes can start lower and elevate to a lower level; e.g. 60 < 75 > 60 or the instructor can decide what will work for the class. Use basic and simple techniques and for the 10-minute test allow the class to use their own techniques as long as they are within the guidelines.

You will by now have gained a more in-depth analysis of heart rate monitoring. The heart plays an extremely important role in our lives as humans and even more as athletes and healthy people. Heart rate monitoring has the stigma attached that it is either for the really fit or for the unhealthy; as you will have discovered, this is far from the truth. By using a heart rate monitor and an application like Heart Zone Training®, training is made simple and more fun. The different sub-max tests can determine your maximum heart rate and allow you to train within the five different zones. Allowing yourself to become familiar with your different heart rates whether it be your ambient heart rate, your delta heart rate, your recovery heart rate, or perhaps the most important of all, your resting heart rate, means not only that you are able to gauge when you are getting sick, but also have useful feedback when determining and monitoring your fitness. Heart rate monitors are cheap and easy tools to use if you know how to use them properly. They provide the accurate feedback that is needed to train correctly, whether your goal is to lose weight, get fit or rehabilitate. Next time you train try measuring your heart rate manually and repeat each time you exercise, because, just like training, monitoring your heart is addictive!

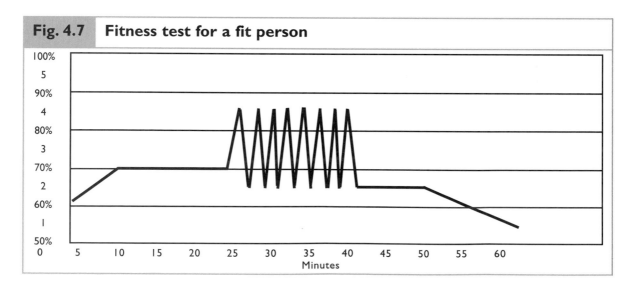

Fig. 4.7 **Fitness test for a fit person**

GENERAL TRAINING ZONES WITHIN A CLASS STRUCTURE

5

In a typical 45-minute class, research has shown that people use up between 300 and 800 calories depending on metabolism. Calories are used by fat metabolism and with glycogen (glucose) expenditure in the muscles, blood and liver. At low intensities a greater percentage of fat is used, but as the intensity increases so does the proportion of glycogen (carbohydrates). The studio training effect will help the body to adapt and develop its potential to burn fat during a class. It is important to replenish glycogen stores after exercise via carbohydrate intake from food and drink.

A balanced training programme will help with weight management, loss or gain from fat stores or muscle masses. This can be achieved through the balance of intensities and times, i.e. fast or slow, easy or hard, long or short. It can sometimes be difficult to understand the principles of calorie expenditure; many people become obsessed with the number of calories versus the length of time spent working out. However it is the instructor's job to educate people into realising that everyone's metabolism increases and will stay higher for a long period of time after leaving the gym.

Instructors should structure all classes based on the class requirements and place them into correct training zones. This can be done by talking to people and finding out their goals. Remember that everyone is an individual; each will respond to the class differently and as such could be overtraining or undertraining unless guided into correct training zones.

When you pedal at different intensities and pedal speeds you will be working in different training zones. We can describe these as 'general training zones' split into four categories. You cannot use '220 – age = maximum heart rate' because this formula has been proved inaccurate in scientific studies, but should use Heart Zone training (as above). Use the RPE scale to calculate intensity and then compare heart rate numbers during the class.

General training zones

Base

Endurance athletes often refer to this lower-intensity training as 'aerobic base training'. It has been shown to be essential for higher-intensity training, as it requires the use of predominantly the fat metabolism as its energy source. Other benefits are flexibility, mobility and enzyme and hormone production.

Typically this level is around 50–70% of maximum heart rate and would be used in a studio-cycling class for the warm-up and warm-down phases, as well as recovery sections or extended classes.

Aerobic

In the aerobic zone the body still has the ability to recycle lactic acid. Lactic acid is a by-product of energy metabolism in the muscles. This is a lower-intensity level where the cardiovascular system is able to supply oxygen to the working muscles quickly enough to prevent the build-up of lactic acid.

Typically this level would be around 70–85% of maximum heart rate and would be used for medium-level challenges within a class structure. The heart as the primary muscle in the body responds with adaptation in this level. The instructor will aim to develop the length of time spent in this zone, especially at the top end just before the anaerobic level. The aerobic threshold is where the primary source of energy is glycogen and fat.

Anaerobic

The anaerobic level is where lactic acid build-up begins to exceed the body's capacity to recycle it. As the increase in performance deteriorates, the feeling known as 'the burn' is experienced. Training by athletes in this zone is primarily to recreate race environments. During a studio-cycling class this level, known, as the 'anaerobic threshold', would be used within intervals or hard sections such as climbing a hill; the primary energy source would be glycogen. No extra fat is burnt, as oxygen is not present.

Typically the levels used in this zone would be 85–95% of maximum heart rate.

Maximal

Maximal heart rate is above the anaerobic threshold where failure comes quickly, such as the end of a sprint or very high resistance used at the peak of a hill. No one should reach their maximum during a 45-minute class; if they do, then something is wrong with the style of teaching. Maximal has no part to play in studio cycling – it is too intense and would render the rider unable to continue properly or with the correct energy stores.

Heart rates could vary from 95–100% of maximum. Energy supplied would be glycogen and, in extreme cases, protein.

Instructor tip:

At the start of a class, discuss the profile and the class goals. For example, if you are going to do a 'threshold class' use analogies such as this story of a marathon runner. 'Jim's aim is to run at the highest possible heart rate for the whole London Marathon. He has trained hard and knows his threshold is around 166 bpm. If he can still maintain this heart rate at the end of the race he knows he will have had the best possible race. He starts off a little lower than 166 bpm, at 158 bpm. This is an easier pace for him as his taper after long, hard training runs means his threshold is high and he is fresh. After 13 miles he is still on track, never going above 166 bpm, although this seems easy too. He is continually holding back. If he goes above this rate he will slow down and not do his best time. At the end of the race lactic acid build-up would mean his heart rate would be much lower, but if the heart rate is sustained he would have done the optimum time for that day. In the class today we are going to train at and around our threshold. We can raise this threshold if we train in multiple zones. This will raise our fat-burning range and create incredible fitness!'

Class breakdown

Each class, whether it be 20 minutes or 1 hour long, has to be broken down into different sections. Each section has an important role in both safety and efficiency within the class environment. There are four main sections to a class which vary in length depending on the length of the class itself.

Section 1a. Warm-up

The role of this section is for the instructor to warm the body up for about 5–10 minutes using resistance and pedalling at speed. The aim is to raise the core temperature of the body without working too hard. A good sign of a warm-up is when excess clothing starts to be removed. The music for the warm-up should be relaxing and appropriate for this section. The heart rate stays at a low ambient, normally in Zone 2. Warmed muscles will contract and release more efficiently, which benefits strength and speed in studio-cycling techniques. Range of movement and mobility around the joints benefits from an efficient warm-up. Connective tissue becomes more pliable, with better fluidity of the synovial fluid inside joints created by higher blood temperature.

The blood temperature is increased as it passes through the muscle. As this happens the quantity of oxygen in the bloodstream is reduced and it is transported into the muscles more readily. Therefore the volume of oxygen to the working muscles will enhance endurance and speed. Zone 2 (60–70% of max) is known as the temperate zone (see Fig. 4.4) It is a well-known fact that in this zone we become more focused and positive, this is because the increased oxygen supply to the brain improves mental alertness and helps us prepare for more intense exercise.

Hormones that regulate energy production are produced. In turn they make carbohydrates and fatty acids available for energy. The body's metabolism within the muscles speeds up approximately 13% along with the core temperature's rise. Each individual will warm up at their own pace and this has to be of concern to the instructor. It will be important to get the relevant feedback to determine that everyone has sufficiently warmed up to move to the next phase of the class. Reasons for poor warm-up could be: hunger, tiredness, lack of fitness, dehydration, stress, temperature or illness.

Section 1b. Mobilisation towards the end of the warm-up

After the warm-up when the core temperature has been raised we move into the section called 'mobilisation'. Mobilisation abbreviated from movement requires basic movement exercises from the upper body to increase mobility and relaxation for when we return to the handlebars. Within reason any exercise using the arms and shoulders, using appropriate music, is sufficient providing the exercises are safe. **This is not stretching**! But will aid a positive warm-up. With cycling the muscle contraction is actively dynamic and the muscles in the lower body move and warm up through their full range. This reduces the need for pre-class stretching. Indeed, if you were to get off the bike and stretch the cooling effect on the muscles would cause you to need another warm-up, taking valuable time away from the rest of the class.

Examples of mobilisation techniques:
• Roll the shoulders.
• Gently swing the arms from side to side.
• Swing the arms back in a backstroke movement.
• Dip the head slowly.
• Turn the head from side to side (see Fig. 5.1).

Section 2. Pre-main set

The role of the pre-main set (see Fig. 5.2), which lasts about 5 minutes, is to elevate the heart rate progressively using a series of short challenges to prepare the body for the main set. These challenges again can comprise of adding resistance and changing the road taking RPE up to 7 or 7.5 maximum for the more advanced cyclists. The music for this part should be distinctly more motivating in some way.

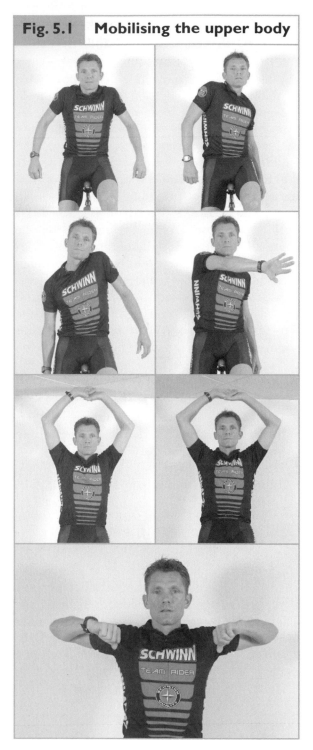

Fig. 5.1 Mobilising the upper body

Section 3. The main set

The main set (see Fig. 5.2) is where the class should spend and develop most of their time. It comprises a variation of challenges suitable for the ability of the group. The music for this section should change once again and be motivational in some way. Most fitness improvements are gained when time in the main set is increased progressively. RPE can reach a maximum of 9.5 depending on the ability of the group and the training zone. However the most common and beneficial classes for the first 2–3 months will be spent in Zone 3 to the mid-point of Zone 4 or anaerobic threshold.

Section 4. Recovery and stretching 5–10 minutes

The aim of the recovery (not cool-down) is to keep the core temperature high but reduce heart rate and intensity progressively to aid effective recovery. Resistance and cadence should be decreased as the group recovers. Music should change once again to be more relaxing and highlight the fact the session is coming to an end.

It is vital now that the circulation gradually recovers to near resting levels. You can see that this should follow a pattern more like a series of steps than a steep line. A more efficient recovery will be to bring the heart rate and leg speeds down in a linear fashion, preventing blood pooling, which can occur if you stop too quickly and blood accumulates in the dilated blood vessels thus preventing efficient venous return. A rapid heart rate that is trying to get the blood to the heart and oxygen to the working muscles will cause dizziness or light-headedness. This is one reason why we are careful not to recover with an elevated body or arms above our heads.

Active recovery increases the speed at which lactic acid is removed from the blood and muscles, and enables a quick recovery from any oxygen debt.

Stretching of the upper body (on the bike) and lower body (off the bike) would follow on after recovery. The upper body stretches can be done while the legs are moving slowly and in control. A consistent upper body routine will include stretches that last for 10–15 seconds or two breaths in and out.

The lower body stretches are extremely important as we have been working concentrically on the bikes. The leg muscles have been contracting and will be shortened. A good and progressive stretch routine will be progressive and cover all the major leg muscle groups, maintaining or even increasing flexibility. A structured routine of lower body and progressive stretches must be implemented. Try to extend the duration of the stretches allowing for at least 15–20 seconds or three long breaths in and out.

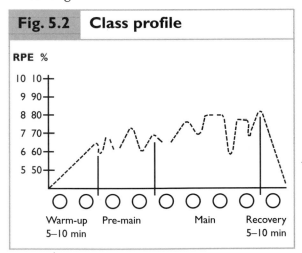

Fig. 5.2 **Class profile**

Do not use the bike to stretch the lower body, keep the stretches safe. By lifting your leg onto the bike you are increasing the chances of an accident and potential injury. Keep it simple.

Another good reason not to use the bike is the maintenance issue. The bottom bracket is incredibly strong when it is moving, but once it is static and you apply external forces such as that of a good hamstring stretch, the lifespan of the bottom bracket will be halved. There are plenty of safe stretches that we can do off the bike.

Above is an example class profile showing each of the four sections. The drops after a particular challenge would be short recovery periods including a drink and towel down. Time for these varies again depending on the ability of the group.

The class environment

Setting the scene

Before the first class an instructor must think how to set the scene.

It's Monday night, 6.30 pm, time for your class; everyone is set up on their bikes waiting for you to start the class. Music on, pedals turn, the journey has begun.

Each person starts and finishes the journey at the same time but they all take different roads. No one is the same, all are individuals, and we can't all ride at exactly the same speed and intensity. None of the bikes are calibrated to the same degree, so we ride against ourselves. This is not a race against anyone; let your class members take energy from those around them, the instructor and the music. Use these things to help motivate you and your class, but let them understand and do it for themselves.

Tell the class, 'Today you train for *you*, forget about work and the stresses of everyday life, leave it all behind; turn the pedals and ride down your road to fitness and health – let's go!'

As you start on your own personal journey you will require dedication and commitment.

Let the philosophies and physical efforts of teaching and training in studio cycling become part of your lifestyle. Work hard and balance intense effort with recovery time, lead your class by example and you will capture the essence of this limitless concept.

Pre class Checks

- ⚲ Welcome pupils, relax them and make them feel at ease.
- ⚲ Advise as to any reasons why they shouldn't take part, mentioned in Health Check.
- ⚲ Bike check.
- ⚲ Level of participants' fitness.

Instructors should remember that complete beginners will spend a large percentage of their class time in the base zone and during their first few classes they will make large improvements to their cardiovascular and respiratory systems. **You must remember to teach to the ability of the class** – you may have a brilliant programme planned for the group but if they are not ready for that intensity or duration you must change it to suit them. You are probably very fit yourself and you may begin to take this for granted, but something particularly easy for you may be extremely difficult for a beginner. It can take 2–3 classes for beginners to actually get used to the bikes and different techniques.

To incorporate progression in your classes you must change intensity and duration over weeks and months.

Fitness elements

Aerobic endurance 70–85%

Your first goal is to build time spent on aerobic endurance. Instructors can use the class profiles and draw progression graphs in the main set to indicate changes in frequency, duration and time within 70–85%. This will vary from individual to individual but the first phase is usually 2–3 months long.

Strength 70+%

Whilst you are in the aerobic endurance phase you will be building strength; however, after the first phase you can add actual strength elements periodically. These will consist of steeper hill climbs, repeated depending on the fitness levels of the class. These hills can be progressive by increasing frequency, intensity and/or duration.

Table 5.1	Class profile chart			
Zone	When and what	% max HR	Time	RPE
Base	= Warm-up+ Recovery Predominantly fat	50-70%	Min/Hr	5-7
Aerobic	= Pre-main+ Main Fat/carbs	70-85%	Min/Hr	7-8.5
Anaerobic	= Main Carbs	85-95%	Min	8.5-9.5
Maximal	= Main Carbs/protein	95-100%	Sec	9.5+

Speed 70+%

Speed is added only after the individuals have been working on the two elements above for a period of normally several months. Of course there is already an element of speed in any mobility activity but the speed element will be added using key sprints.

Power 80+%

> **Instructor tip:**
>
> By including these simple progressive elements your classes will seem more varied which will ensure that your clients keep returning.

Power is a combination of strength and speed; therefore it is a very advanced element to add. It is explosive and will be used only occasionally during the programme when the

> **Instructor training tip:**
>
> The following different techniques are sometimes demonstrated in different levels of class:
>
> - Intervals – increase resistance/intensity or leg speed for a set time.
> - Pyramid training – building pace with time or just time then returning to beginning.
> - Time trial with visualisation – using imagery combined with focus and concentration, get the group from A to B in the fastest time. Everyone is a winner!
> - Pace line intervals – work as a group with one person in the lead for a set time before dropping to the back.
> - Sprint intervals – imagine a race against others to the line. Everyone is a winner!
> - Running intervals – as intervals but in running position 2, out of the saddle.

class has been training for over 2 months. Pick key music with a definite rhythm that speeds up quickly. This will only ever be done with high resistance.

The four fitness elements above will have all these qualities in common and more:
- Flexibility
- Mobility
- Dedication
- Motivation
- Mental strength.

Ride the studio-cycling bike on the journey

'We start the journey on our bike out on the open road. As with all bike rides the road doesn't stay the same, it goes up hills, down hills, round corners; there are fast sections with the wind behind you and tough sections when the wind is against you.' Your programme must be ever changing to the needs of the class.

On the road we have two types of terrain – **flat roads** and **hills**.

Flat roads can be ridden with little or no resistance to start with. There will be times when resistance can be used but generally a flat road would be associated with a higher cadence or revolutions per minute (rpm). As strength is developed it will be possible to add resistance and keep a higher cadence. This type of riding can be associated with racing on a flat road.

Hills (or climbing) are simulated by adding resistance; it gets harder to pedal and our cadence slows down. As the road climbs and becomes too hard to stay seated it is possible to rise and *climb* out of the saddle.

Warm up gently

Use the music carefully to help you start at the correct cadence with low resistance on the flywheel. Studio cycling has an advantage over other forms of exercise because it is load-bearing (no impact). You can keep the heart rate relatively low to start with while you spin the pedals and warm up the legs and the rest of the body. After 5–10 minutes the class can progressively add resistance and or speed up their pedalling to raise the heart rate gradually. A well warmed-up class will be able to handle a higher intensity programme.

Recovery

After a tough class it is very important to allow gradual recovery by easing resistance and/or slowing down the pedalling action. This will allow the heart rate to drop and the blood to return from the extremities back to the heart and brain. It is also helpful with speeding up recovery times.

Lactate can build up during intense exercise; a gentle warm-down will reduce blood pooling in the muscles.

A safe class!

It is of paramount importance to let the class train at their own individual level. In every class there will be novice and experienced together. This should not be a problem provided the instructor is aware of everyone's background and observes the individuals throughout the class.

It is when a beginner has their first ride that you must make sure the class structure enables them to progress to the more advanced techniques at their own pace. You cannot run before you walk.

Make sure you are hydrated before the class and have eaten no less than two hours before-hand. Stay at your own pace!

Things to remember when teaching your first studio-cycling class:

Class members start to arrive
1 Introduce yourself

2 Ask members' names, goals and history of exercise
3 Ensure bags go in changing room
4 Set up new members on bikes
5 Do they have water and towels?

Warm-up
1 Don't turn music on till ready
2 Discuss with class where they are with training programme, e.g. Week 3 etc.
3 Biomechanics
4 Cadence check
5 Heart rate check
6 Upper body de-stress mobility
7 Feedbacks × 3

Pre-main set – elevate heart rate
1 Biomechanics
2 Be aware of level of individuals
3 Use 2–5 short, progressive efforts
4 Feedback × 3

Main set to include 3 elements
1 Employ fun motivation and high energy using your personality and the music
2 Proceed with mental training – visualisation, relaxation, focusing and concentration to be added progressively as group become more experienced.
3 Create training programme by increasing frequency, intensities and time in main sets as group become fitter and more experienced, using the 4-weekly cycles.

Recovery
1 Reduce intensity and pedal speed (cadence)
2 Slow breathing
3 Stretch upper body on bike
4 Stretch lower body off bike

After class
1 Obtain feedback from group (music, intensity, techniques, enjoyment etc.)
2 Book future classes
3 Be last to leave.

Music

Music gives studio cycling passion!

The music rules

Rule 1. Motivation and how to choose the right music

Use music to motivate you: if you are not motivated it will rub off on the class. Ask advice if you have a really bad taste in music. Don't forget that music is individually subjective – one person could love it and another hate it.

Rule 2. Variety

One of the great things about studio cycling is that you can use almost any type of music to ride to. If it fits and it works, use it. Classical music probably has the broadest range of bpm. Listen to music with a different ear, find something inspirational in it. Often it is just a spark that makes the hairs on the back of your neck stand up. (See Table 5.2 for general music speeds.)

Rule 3. Music Speeds/bpm/cadence/rhythm

Always know the speed of the music and give the class the guidelines. You can use music to help you ride at the correct pace, by choosing tracks with the rhythm or beats per minute that fits the leg speed or cadence you want to ride at. The right music at the right time will help the instructor control a class, through relaxation, stimulation and motivation. Check the beat of your selected music for 15 seconds and multiply by 4, this will give you the beats per minute (bpm).

If you wish to have your class members ride to the beat of the music you can do a cadence check which will give them the revolutions per minute (rpm). Bring the knee to the elbow on one side, count how many times the elbow touches the knee in 15 seconds and multiply by 4. You can get the class to ride to the beat or off the beat depending on the technique you choose. Pace changes can be worked around the beat of the music.

> **Technique guidelines for rpm**
> (use this when choosing your music – see below):
>
> Seated flat, 70–100 rpm
> Standing flat, 60–90 rpm
> Seated climbs, 50–70 rpm
> Standing climbs, 60–70 rpm
> Combination flat, 70–90 rpm
> Combination hill, 50–60 rpm

Rule 4. Feedback

Find out from the class members whether they liked the music, ask them how it made them feel! This will help you build new music for new classes.

Rule 5. Expense

Don't buy too much of your own music; it will get scratched, lost and ruined after too many classes with only one CD player. It can become very expensive too if you are always looking for new music to give your classes a little extra.

Rule 6. Motivation

Music helps you to cut out distractions, enabling the class to focus; but also use it to inspire and motivate. Music can tell a story, or it can create feelings. For example, a piece of music can make you happy if it reminds you of a time in your life or a person you love. Music inspires feelings that can give an emotional ride as well as a physical one. If someone is high on the music they could give that extra 10 per cent in the class.

However, your music must inspire you so you can inspire the group – but you must draw a line. Use music that reinforces the particular part of the programme you are teaching. Your favourite Guns 'n' Roses album would not be suitable for a 45-minute beginners' class!

Whilst the music is your own personal choice, it must fit certain elements of the class, for example:
- Warm-up – relaxing/motivating
- Pre-main set – slightly more motivating, increase intensity
- Main set – different motivational music
- Recovery – relaxing and highlighting session near to the end, decrease the volume.

Planning studio-cycling signs and maps

Planning your class is vital, from arranging the music (as already discussed), to planning the actual style of road that you wish to ride. The small symbols (see Fig. 5.5) are used to identify the different styles of roads you are riding. Each type of road (seated flat, climbs etc.) has a special map which is instantly recognisable. You can design your class programme to

Instructor tip:
- Create a library of music with other instructors.
- If the class is inexperienced at counting cadence let them follow or mimic your leg speed.
- Start to 'feel' the cadence and know the rpms instinctively.
- What music inspires one person won't necessarily help another.
- Invite class members to bring music in for you to listen and ride to.

incorporate different challenges and use the maps to help you. See Chapter 6, Further Assistance For Instructors.

By compiling the signs you can create an imaginative ride that will be fun and challenging, but remember they are not set in stone, so use them as guidelines only. Do not forget that in your classes there will be all levels and abilities; you must be sensitive to their needs.

Create maps for each class and don't use the same map all the time. As you will find out, you can ride to a piece of music differently each time it's played as there are many beats and

Table 5.2	General music speeds and applications	
Type of music	Technique/terrain to the beat	Approximate beats per minute
World	Flats and hills	80 – 120
Ambient	Flats and hills	80 – 120
Popular	Flats and hills	60 – 140
Classical	All	50 – 200
Trance	Flats (half time) and hills (half time)	130 – 160
House	Fast flat and hills	120 – 140
Drum and Bases	Hills (half time)	150 – 180
Blues	Hills and flats	60 – 110
Chill-out	Flats and hills	80 – 120

rhythms to find; however, this will not inspire the class. You can come up with your own maps and signs because you are the only one who needs to understand them.

> **Instructor tip:**
>
> Have a CD changer that can hold five or more CDs. This will stop you breaking the flow of your class when changing one to the other as well as preventing damage from sweat when handling them.
>
> In many countries now there are licensing laws to protect the artist. It is very important to have a Public Performance licence (PPL), because playing copied recordings during your class can be breaking the law, and it carries a hefty fine. The licence isn't as expensive as a £3,000+ fine.

How to run a 45-minute class

If you are an instructor teaching your classes in a health club or gym you have to be flexible about their needs. Classes therefore need to be broken down into different levels, so as to cater for all abilities. Give the classes names:

A Class – Beginners/newcomers/induction class
B Class – Intermediate/middle pack
C Class – Advanced/competition class.

Each group learns basics first and then moves on to more advanced ideas later when it is ready.

Type A class

A type A class is for complete beginners to studio cycling.

Fig. 5.5	Studio cycling map signs
Seated flat 80–120 rpm	
Seated climb 60–80 rpm	
Standing flat or running 80–120 rpm	
Standing climb 60–80 rpm	
Combinations – flats (jumping) 60–110 rpm	
Combination – hills (jumping) 60–80 rpm	
Stepping 60–120 rpm	
Sprinting – flats and hills >110 rpm	
Walk/jog/run Below beat/to the beat/above the beat	
Walk/jog/run/sprint Faster than above the beat (110 max rpm)	

Type A class highlights

🚲 Safety
🚲 Set-up
🚲 Warm-up
🚲 Introduction to hand positions
🚲 Introduction to basic techniques (flats and hills, seated and standing)
🚲 Recovery class
See Table 5.3.

Key Points

- Remind clients to train at their own level.
- Encourage them to challenge themselves.
- Keep an eye on your class.
- Be positive – give clear and audible instructions.
- Reinforce deep breathing and relaxation.
- Lead and motivate, don't be scared to try new moves but remember, 'simplicity' is best.
- Stick to the **map**.
- Challenge with music and light visualisation.
- Cool down and stretch off the bike.
- Clean the bikes down.
- Advise recommended 2–3 classes per week.
- Arrange to see them the next time and thank them for coming!

Instructor tip:

If you structure these classes then beginners and newcomers will feel more at ease and not think that studio cycling is just for the really fit! These people are journey people and will follow you as the instructor because they like to think you are looking after them. They will come back again and again.

- Prepare your music and maps in advance.
- Arrive early.
- Follow your class booking instructions.
- Check all bikes for functionality and cleanliness.
- Check sound system and key your first track.
- Say 'hello' to everyone and make eye contact.
- Use experienced studio cyclists to help with initial set-up of bikes or take control: 'No one is to pedal until I say!'
- Remind them – 'No towel or water, no class!'

Type B class

A type B class is for clients in their fourth or more class and it will introduce basic mind/body principles and encourage them to use heart rate monitoring.

Type B class highlights

- Less talking (because the group understands basic techniques and is becoming more focused)
- Warm-up/cool-down and full stretch
- Emphasis on senses and visualisation of the road
- Focusing
- Concentration
- Technique and biomechanics emphasis
- Main set (low and high end endurance, hills)
- Introduction to combinations if class is ready
- Heart rate checks and descriptions
- Recovery class
- Interesting map
- Visual observations of group during class and suggestions made in appropriate areas

See Table 5.4.

Type C class

Type C classes are for intermediate-level studio cyclists who have been training consistently 2–3 times a week for 6+ weeks and are ready to add harder techniques and strengthen their minds.

Type C class highlights

- Again, less talking (group is becoming more focused and familiar with basic techniques)
- Warm-up/cool-down/full stretch
- Strong visualisation

Table 5.3	A class structure sheet (beginner)	
Things to remember	**Key points:**	
Learn names Music Sound system Bikes/other equipment	Technique Coaching points Observation Pick profile/signs to match class levels Recommend other classes in the week RPE scale (don't discuss Heart Rate until B Class)	
Class part	**Elements**	**Notes**
Before class	Safety	Check area for bags, power cables. Ensure towels and water are accessible.
	Bike set-up	Use quick fit bike set-up to be taught from your bike. Give visual and verbal demos and look for obvious set-up problems. Get class to interact during bike set-up.
Warm-up RPE 5–7	Music rhythm	Play first track, to highlight warm-up. Participants should be relaxed and comfortable and look for bike set-up problems. Start pedalling on a flat road 80–120 rpm. Riders choose leg speeds at their *own* rhythm.
	Hand positions	Explain hand positions on bike and their uses. To be used for variety, posture and introduction of visualisation.
	Start visualisation	Ask group to close eyes if they want to, and imagine a place that is familiar to them in a nice environment using positive suggestions with a goal at the end. 80–120 rpm.
	Basic sitting	Participants should sit towards back of saddle, lengthen spine, relax elbows and shoulders, have head in a neutral position, knees over toes and a loose grip on handlebars. Resistance to be added gradually and chosen by them. Hands in position: narrow or wide.
	Basic standing	Group to be adding sufficient resistance that it's hard to pedal sitting down, hands in position: standing climb, one smooth movement standing out of saddle, hips over middle of bike, saddle tapping bottom, loosen grip, transfer weight through pedals, nose crossing centre line. 60–80 rpm. Only to be taught if group is ready. Emphasise that more rather than less resistance makes it easier to

		stand. This is only a short taster for the class to teach technique, and also a good way of generating heat in the body for the warm-up although not designed to raise the heart rate too much.
	Mobilisation (upper)	Upper body movement exercises designed to mobilise upper body ready for main sets. Not stretching.
Pre-main RPE 7–8.5	Other challenges Easy flats or steady hills	Designed to elevate heart rate gradually by adding resistance and prepare the body for following challenges in the main set. Examples include seated or standing climbs but designed to suit the ability of the group. Look for tension and other problems within the group; highlighting, relaxing and specific coaching points for each challenge. Music to be more motivating to highlight different part of class.
	Peddling techniques (biomechanics)	Explained to enhance muscle balance, pedalling efficiency and injury prevention. Coached by breaking down the terms 'push forwards and down, pull back and up' using relative terms such as 'scraping the foot' etc.
Main RPE 7–8.5	Other challenges (RPE)	Main part of class still designed to suit the ability of group and is high energy, fun and motivating. Pedalling speeds not suggested to enable beginner group to ride at own pace.
	Flats and hills (seated and standing)	Challenges to include seated and standing climbs and downhills, aiming to keep effort levels at a peak. For downhills ensure group bend from the hips, change hand position to narrow or wide or aerodynamic and go as low as they feel comfortable with reduced resistance, watching for excess speed – maximum 110–120 rpm. Using RPE scale to gauge intensities. Observation for technique and how group are coping is essential. Music to change once again to highlight different part of class and challenges.
Recovery RPE 7–5	Upper body stretch (on bike)	After main set music changes to highlight recovery; upper body stretches done on bike to include biceps, triceps, upper back, chest, neck.
	Lower body stretch (off bike)	Get group off bikes; lower body stretches to include hip flexors, backside, hamstrings, quadriceps, upper and lower calf. Stretches done off bike to be more specific with technique and highlight a separate part of the class, which is very important
	Clean bikes	Group to wipe bikes down.

Fig. 5.6   A class profile (example)

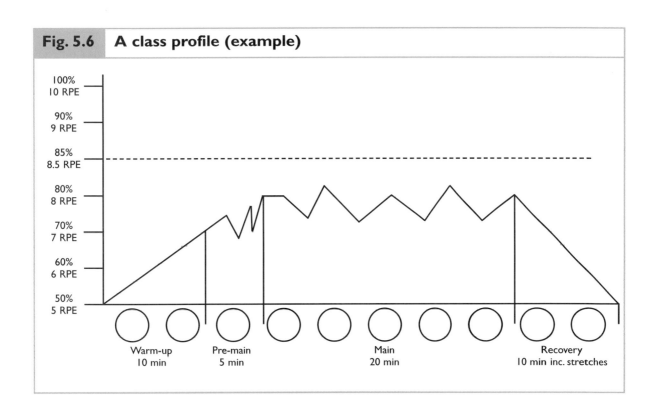

| Warm-up 10 min | Pre-main 5 min | Main 20 min | Recovery 10 min inc. stretches |

Table 5.4   B class structure sheet (beginner to intermediate level)

Things to remember	Key Points
Names A goal for everyone Music Sound system Bikes/other equipment	Technique Coaching points Observation Less talking Pace change Intro to new techniques Profile/signs Introduce the training progamme

Class part	Elements	Notes
Before class	Safety	**As A class** Check area for bags, power cables. Ensure towels and water are accessible.
	Bike set-up	Use quick fit bike set-up, to be taught from your bike. Give visual and verbal demos and look for obvious set-up problems. Get class to interact during bike set-up.

		As A Class
Warm-up RPE 5-7	Music rhythm	Play first track to highlight warm-up. Participants should be relaxed and comfortable and look for bike set-up problems.
	Hand positions	Explain hand positions on bike and their uses. To be used for variety, posture and introduction of visualisation.
		Ask group to close eyes if they want to, and imagine a place that is familiar to them in a nice environment using positive suggestions with a goal at the end.
	Start visualisation, focus and concentration Basic sitting	Participants should sit towards back of saddle, lengthen spine, relax elbows and shoulders, have head in a neutral position, knees over toes and a loose grip on handlebars. Resistance to be added gradually and chosen by them. Hands in position; narrow or wide.
	Mobilisation (upper)	Upper body movement exercises designed to mobilise and de-stress upper body ready for pre- and main sets. This is not stretching.
Pre-main RPE 6-7.5	Basic standing or simple other challenges	As A Class but add intensity and frequency of spikes to 75/80% depending on level of fitness of class members. Group to be adding sufficient resistance so that it is hard to pedal sitting down, hands in position: standing climb, one smooth movement standing out of saddle, hips over middle of bike, saddle tapping bottom, loosen grip, transfer weight through pedals, nose crossing centre line. Only to be taught if group are ready. Emphasise that more rather than less resistance makes it easier to stand.
	Pedalling techniques (biomechanics)	Vary emphasis of pedal action biomechanics. Designed to elevate heart rate gradually by adding resistance and prepare the body for following challenges in the main set. Examples include seated or standing climbs, all designed to suit the ability of the group. Look for tension and other problems within the group; highlighting, relaxing and specific coaching points for each challenge. Music to be more motivating to highlight different part of class. Explained to enhance muscle balance, pedalling efficiency and injury prevention. Coached by breaking down the terms 'push forwards and down, pull back and up' using relative terms such as scraping the foot etc.

	Pace change/ cadence count	Walk – below beat; jog – to the beat; run – above the beat.
Main RPE 7–8.5	Other challenges (RPE)	Main part of class still designed to suit the ability of group and is high energy, fun and motivating. Pedalling speeds not suggested to enable beginner group to ride at own pace. Challenges to include seated and standing climbs and downhills aiming to keep effort levels at a peak. For downhills ensure group bend from the hips, change hand position to an aero position or narrow or wide, go as low as class feels comfortable with reduced resistance, watching for excess speed. 110–120 rpm maximum.
	Introduce Heart Rate Monitoring	Using RPE scale and heart rate to gauge intensities. Use manual 6-second method or HRMs if the class members have them. Observation for technique and how group are coping is essential. Music to change once again to highlight different part of class and challenges.
	Intro to combinations/ jumps (in–out of saddle) Optional depending on level of class	Combination/jumping rhythm 4, 8, or 16 beat, in one smooth movement, hands in wide position, relax upper body, use the legs to support the body, don't lock the legs, keep a natural bend at the hips.
Low end endurance	Flat road 80–120 rpm 65–75%	
Recovery RPE 7–5	Upper body stretch (on bike)	After main set music changes to highlight recovery and upper body stretches done on bike to include biceps, triceps, upper back, chest, neck.
	Lower body stretch (off bike)	Get group off bikes; lower body stretches to include hip flexors, backsides, hamstrings, quadriceps, upper and lower calf. Stretches done off bike to be more specific with technique and highlight a separate part of the class, which is very important. **Be progressive with stretches**
	Clean bikes	Group to wipe bikes down.

Notes: 1 Teach to the level of the class.
2 Progress the intensity and time gradually each class.
3 Keep it simple, teach the basics.

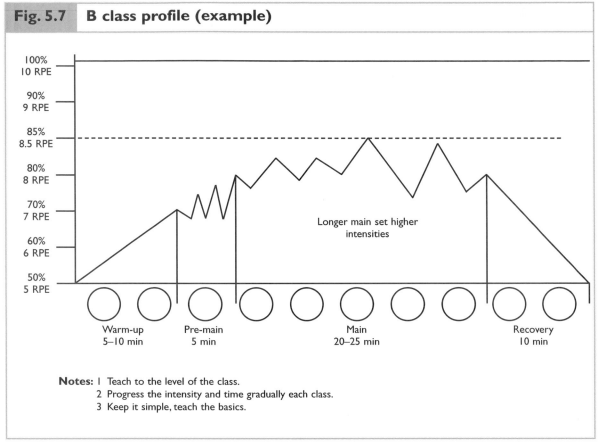

Fig. 5.7   B class profile (example)

Warm-up
5–10 min

Pre-main
5 min

Main
20–25 min

Recovery
10 min

Longer main set higher intensities

Notes: 1 Teach to the level of the class.
2 Progress the intensity and time gradually each class.
3 Keep it simple, teach the basics.

🚲 Goal-setting before and during
🚲 Competition classes (not in every class)
🚲 Low and high end endurance sets
🚲 Recovery class
🚲 Combinations/jumps (not in every class)
🚲 Intensive and extensive intervals (not in every class)
🚲 Hills
🚲 Short sprints (not in every class)
🚲 Eye contact
🚲 Visual observations of group to ensure correct posture and technique
See Table 5.5.

Notes: 1 Teach to the level of the class.
2 Progress the intensity, time and type of technique gradually.

3 Challenge the class to stay longer periods at 85%.
4 Add anaerobic spikes with recovery between work-outs after 2–3 months but not in every class.

Something for you to try: create a map for your first 45-minute class

Use Table 5.6 and Fig 5.9 to help you create a class plan. List the music that you will choose for each piece of the road.

Table 5.5	C class structure sheet (intermediate to advanced level)	
Things to remember	**Key Points**	
Name/goal/background of members Music Sound system Bikes/other equipment	Training programme Technique Coaching points Observation Fewer commands, more focus Pace change, intensity	
Class part	**Elements**	**Notes**
Before class	Safety Bike set-up	**As Classes A and B** Check area for bags, power cables. Ensure towels and water are accessible. Look for visual set-up problems or solutions. Get class to interact during their own bike set-up
Warm-up RPE 5–7	Heart rate check	**As Classes A and B** First track playing used to highlight warm-up. Participants should be relaxed and comfortable and look for bike set-up problems.
	Goal-setting – before, during and after	Ask group to close eyes if they want to, and imagine a place that is **motivating** to them in a **challenging** environment using positive suggestions with a goal at the end. Participants should sit towards back of saddle, lengthen spine, relax elbows and shoulders, have head in a neutral position, knees over toes and a loose grip on handlebars. Resistance to be added gradually and chosen by them. Hands in position 1 or 2.
	Mobilisation (upper)	Upper body movement exercises designed to mobilise upper body ready for main sets. Not stretching.
Pre-main RPE 7–8.5	Standing flats Hills seated and standing Other challenges	**As Classes A and B but add frequency of spikes to 85%** **Vary emphasis of pedal action biomechanics, combinations etc.** Designed to elevate heart rate gradually by adding resistance and prepare the body for following challenges in the main set. Examples include seated or standing climbs, designed to suit the ability of the group. Look for tension and other problems within the group; highlighting relaxing and specific coaching points for each challenge. Music to be more motivating to highlight different part of class.

	Pedalling techniques (biomechanics) Pace change	Explained to enhance muscle balance, pedalling efficiency and injury prevention. Coached by breaking down the terms 'push forwards and down, pull back and up' using relative terms such as 'scraping the foot' etc. Walk – below beat; Jog – to the beat; Run – above the beat.
Main RPE 7–8.5	Other challenges (RPE) - Combinations flat or hills/jumps and stepping Optional depending on level of class Measure recovery heart rates Eye contact Pace, lines, formats Sprints	Main part of class still designed to suit the ability of group and is high energy, fun and motivating. Challenges to include seated flats and climbs, standing climbs and downhills aiming to keep effort levels at a peak; go as low as class feels comfortable with reduced resistance, watching for excess speed. Combination rhythm 4, 8, or 16 beat, in one smooth movement. Use stepping for recoveries – out of saddle to 1, 2, 4, 8 beats. Designed to maintain heart rate but mentally recover class members. Build teams and emphasise rhythm. Give manual and heart monitor recovery tests after main intervals. Measure for 1 or 2 minutes. Repeat every 3–4 weeks. Use to aid motivation of individual and class. Use cycling techniques and names to motivate and split into individual intensities. Split into groups, pairs, individuals etc With resistance complete sprints for 10–15 seconds – use goals e.g. race finish line etc. Max rpm is 110 bpm high resistance.
Recovery RPE 7–5	Upper body stretch (on bike) Lower body stretch (off bike) Clean bikes	After main set music changes to highlight recovery, and upper body stretches done on bike to include biceps, triceps, upper back, chest, neck. Get group off bikes; lower body stretches to include hip flexors, backside, hamstrings, quadriceps, upper and lower calf. Stretches done off bike to be more specific with technique and highlight a separate part of the class, which is very important. Be progressive with stretches. Incorporate longer, slower, deeper stretches periodically to show class members stretches they can do on their own. Group to wipe bikes down.

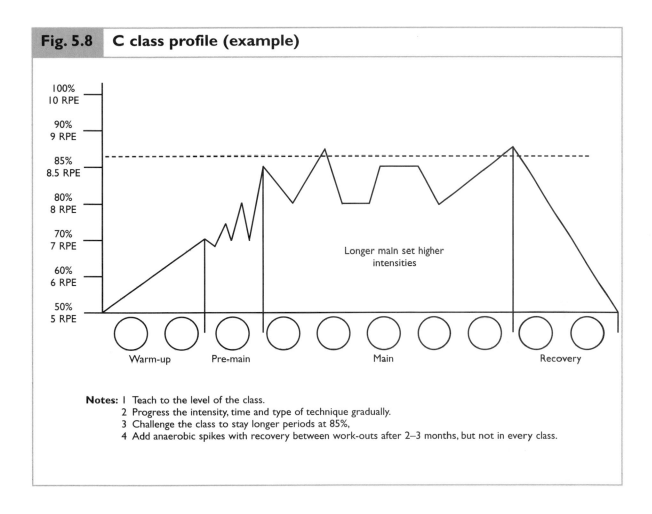

Fig. 5.8 | C class profile (example)

Notes: 1 Teach to the level of the class.
2 Progress the intensity, time and type of technique gradually.
3 Challenge the class to stay longer periods at 85%,
4 Add anaerobic spikes with recovery between work-outs after 2–3 months, but not in every class.

Table 5.6	List of music tracks for 45-minute class	
	Track	Time
1		
2		
3		
4		
5		
6		
7		
8		

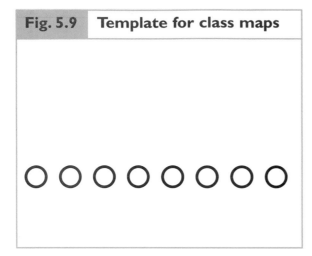

Fig. 5.9 — Template for class maps

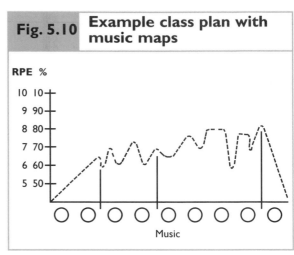

Fig. 5.10 — Example class plan with music maps

Instructor tip:

During a class you may pick up on an individual who is doing something wrong and you need to correct it. Unless you know the person well it is not advisable to make a suggestion to that individual in front of the group as they may feel silly or take the comment personally. You should make your comment to the whole group, the people who are using the right technique will hear you and not change and the person you are actually talking to will, it is hoped, change. There is nothing wrong with emphasising good technique to everyone.

Create a map for an advanced class

Figure 5.10 is an example class plan that you can design using your music maps, showing the different types of road in relation to intensity. (Note: aerobic challenges are shown by peaks and recovery breaks by drops.)

Once you have designed your class programme, you will be able to note it on a small piece of paper kept next to your bike from which to teach. Of course, you do not have to plan your class in this way; just find a method that works for you.

The plan that you have designed will have the appropriate music map the section of class (warm-up, pre-main etc.), track name or number, disc number of CD, and the length of the track (see Table 5.7). You should position it so that you are able to glance down and immediately recognise where you are in your class and what is coming next.

Remember, you may have a brilliant class programme planned out with all your new ideas and challenges, but you *must* teach to the ability of the group and be willing to change your class content on the spot, especially if the group is not ready for your ideas.

Table 5.7	Example class plan chart	
WARM-UP		
Track	Track No.	Disc no.
Enya	3 and 4	1
Deep Forest	2	2
PRE-MAIN		
Ministry	2	3
	4	
	6	
MAIN		
James Brown	2	4
	4	
Kiss in Ibiza	1	5
		3
RECOVERY		
Café del Mar	1 and 2	6

Muscles and flexibility for studio cycling

Stretching so that the body becomes relaxed, loose and flexible will be an integral part of your class programme. How many times have we seen sports people break down because of injury? How many times is it because of neglected warm-up and flexibility? Cycling hard will tighten up different muscle groups. Tight muscles will impede performance and increase risk of injury. In order to put together a correct stretch routine we need to know a little about the muscles and how they work when cycling.

There are three types of muscles; the smooth muscle, cardiac muscle and skeletal muscle. We need to think only about the skeletal muscle, also known as striated or striped muscle. Muscles are made up of connective tissue or fascia and bundles of muscle cells or muscle fibre, and the muscle cell is seen to be composed of small components called muscle fibrils (meaning 'little fibres'). These lie in parallel. The fibrils are made up of smaller components called myofilaments, which are regularly aligned. Myofilaments are chains of protein molecules. The striated appearance is due to the presence of two types of myofilament, actin and myosin. When the muscle contracts, the actin filaments move between the myosin filaments. As a consequence, the myofibrils shorten and thicken. The connective tissue surrounding the muscle extends and is continuous with the muscle's tendon. When the muscle contracts it produces force, which affects the origin and insertion of a muscle equally, but in opposite directions.

The muscles of the body have very different shapes. When analysing movement a muscle's force of contraction depends on its contracted length as compared to its length at rest. Dynamic work means that the origin and insertion of a muscle are forcefully affected by changes in muscle length. If the muscle force causes the origin and insertion to move towards each other, this means that the muscle is working concentrically (the muscle is shortened and contracted) as with the correct pedalling action in studio-cycling classes. If the forces exerted while the origin and insertion are receding from each other (i.e. the muscle tries to stop movement in the joint), the muscle is working eccentrically; although the muscle tries to shorten, it is actually lengthened by external forces, i.e. the flywheel, if there is not enough resistance. Anyone trying to spin too fast with too little resistance is working eccentrically.

When the muscles contract without any movement taking place in the joint the muscle is working statically or isometrically. This should never occur in a class because the flywheel should never stop unless we add resistance or the brake.

When the muscle cells stretch, so do the muscle spindles (nerve cells). If the muscle stretches too much, risking injury, the muscle spindle sends a signal to the muscle to contract, which prevents the muscle from being injured. This protective mechanism works for sudden stretches, but permits voluntary stretches that are not too sudden.

All these systems can break down, with a greater chance of injury, if the warm-up and recovery parts of the class are not adhered to along with good stretch routines.

Elastic stretching or mobility exercises have nothing to do with stretching the muscles, although this method has been used with some success by dancers for many years. Such exercises should be used only when warming up. Progressive stretches are designed to lengthen the muscle groups quickly, in turn increasing the range of motion in the joints. Both kinds of stretch are valuable in our classes but we should use the elastic stretches before the class and the other progressive stretches at the end when we are very warm.

Studies have shown that if the muscle contracts first and then stretches slowly it can extend a little further. This method of Facilitated or PNF (Proprioceptive Neuromuscular Facilitating) stretches could be used after the class on the longer stretch routine days, when you show the class the longer, slower, deeper stretches they can and should do on their own.

Areas that will be stretched in a studio-cycling class routine are: chest, shoulders, triceps, upper and lower back, neck, quadriceps, backside, hamstrings, calves, inner thigh, hip flexors. Some areas are exercised more than others but in order to achieve a balance you should spend appropriate time on each area. Remember, when students come to train they bring with them the baggage of their lifestyle in the shape of many different stresses, and to miss out an area may cause them an imbalance.

Muscles must be in a state of readiness for work, so we have to be careful what type of stretching we do and when we do it. This is why it is important to warm up on the bike before cycling hard and to do passive and PNF stretching only towards the end of a class or, in some cases, when the muscles have been properly warmed.

Muscles can become knotted, inefficient and unable to contract properly; when this happens other muscle groups take over and injury is not far away. Use elastic and passive stretching carefully to keep muscles fresh and ready for the next class.

Please note that no stretching for the lower body should be done on the bike, as it can be dangerous and place unnecessary strain on the body as well as wear and tear on parts of the bike, for example the bearings, handlebars, and other components.

For how long should we stretch?

After a class it is normal to spend at least 5 minutes stretching; however, this may not be long enough to stretch each area sufficiently, therefore advise members to complete their own stretching routine in their own time after the class.

Basic elastic/mobility stretch routine – during warm-up

You can use these or make up your own, but keep them simple!

- Shoulder movements: rotate your arms/elbows in a slow circular motion whilst pedalling
- Arm swings: swing each arm forwards and reverse several times and alternate this
- Upright arm pull downs: straighten and bend arms above the head and down to the shoulders
- Chest curls and combination of the two: elbows up at chest height, hands straight above them, bring them in and out rhythmically
- Centring: breathe in through the nose and lift

your arms straight up above your head, then in a circular motion to the side bring your arms round and down whilst breathing out through the mouth and contracting your abdominals; repeat 5–10 times.

Basic passive stretch routine – after the class

Upper body (on bike)

Upper body stretches can be done carefully on the bike. Hold each stretch for 10–15 seconds, or approximately two breaths in and two breaths out. It is possible to keep the legs moving as long as they are slow and controlled. This aids recovery and prevents blood pooling. Maintain correct posture with active abdominals. See Fig. 5.11.

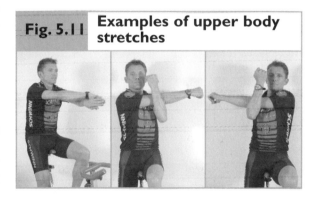

Fig. 5.11 Examples of upper body stretches

Shoulders/Trapezius

Sit on the bike and pedal slowly. Take your arms straight out to the front and press your hands lightly together. Roll your shoulders slightly forwards. See Fig. 5.12.

Fig. 5.12 Shoulder stretch

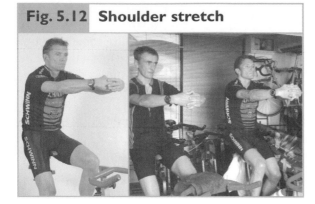

Deltoid

Sit on the bike and pedal slowly. Take your arms behind your body and clasp your hands lightly. Push your hands away from your back. To increase the stretch let your head come slowly forward.

Chest/Pectoralis major

Sit on the bike and pedal slowly. Take your hands behind you and gently press your hands into your back, with your elbows moving towards each other.

Fig. 5.13 Deltoid stretch

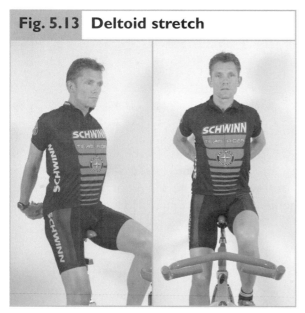

Triceps and Teres major

Sit on the bike and pedal slowly. Stretch one arm to the ceiling, bend it at the elbow and take the hand down the centre of your back. Gently rest the weight of your other arm onto the raised elbow to increase the stretch of the tricep. Repeat on both arms.

Fig. 5.14 Tricep stretch

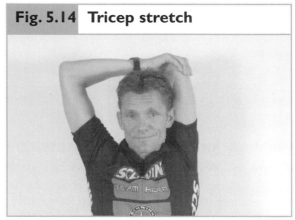

Neck/Sterno-cleido-mastoid

Sit on the bike and pedal slowly. Let your head gently come forwards. Extend your arms down on each side towards the floor. Feel the stretch across the neck. Roll or turn your head to one side and hold it there for five seconds then gently roll or turn round to the other side.

Fig. 5.15 Neck stretch

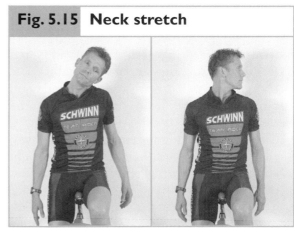

Lower body (off bike)

Lower body stretches should be performed carefully off the bike. Hold each stretch for 15–20 seconds, or approximately three breaths in and three breaths out.

Quadriceps/rectus femoris

Stand by the bike and support yourself with one hand on the bike. Bring the heal of one foot to your backside and hold towards your backside. Bend your supporting leg slightly. To increase the stretch press the knee of your supporting leg towards the floor, and try carefully bringing the same knee gently backwards under the hips (see Fig. 5.16).

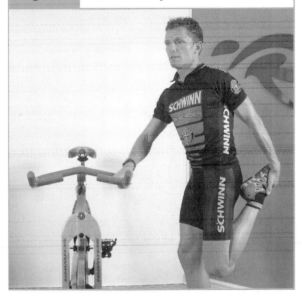

Fig. 5.16 **Quadriceps stretch**

Gluteus maximus

1/ Bring your knee up towards your chest, supporting your knee underneath. Lift until you can feel the stretch. (At the same time rotate the foot both ways to loosen off the Achilles and calf muscle.) Keep your supporting leg slightly bent.

2/ Bend your supporting leg and carefully place the opposite foot across the thigh. Increase the stretch into the buttocks by pushing your backside gently backwards; allowing the body to come forwards with a neutral back. Women love this stretch, however some men can find this difficult with some discomfort, especially in the knee that is up. Focus on slow breathing and progressively increasing the stretch without any feeling in the knee (see Fig. 5.17).

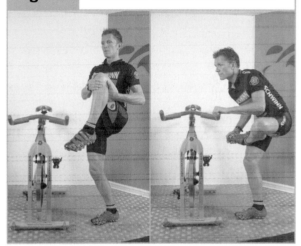

Fig. 5.17 **Gluteus maximus stetch**

Elastic stretch: calves/achilles tendon

Use a solid object such as a wall or the bike to support and push against. Place one leg backwards and press the heel of that foot into the ground to feel a light stretch. To deepen the stretch, let your hips come forwards, dropping the front knee at the same time. For those who find this not a deep enough stretch, they can use the back bar of the bike by raising the front toes up which will increase the stretch. If the muscles become tight, back off slightly to ensure you do not over stretch the muscle.

Do this stretch after the previous calf stretch. Bring the rear leg half way in and drop the knee to increase the stretch.

Fig. 5.18 Calf stretches

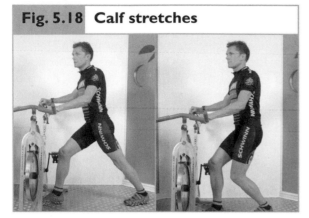

Hamstrings/bicep femoris and
semitendinosus and semimembranosus

Straighten your front leg and bend your rear
leg. Place your hands on the quadriceps of the
rear bent leg and slowly bring your hips back
away from the front heel to increase the stretch.
Bend forwards with your back maintaining a
neutral position for 10–15 seconds (see fig.
5.19). You can then flex your front toes up for
another 10 seconds to lengthen the stretch time
and add an extra calf stretch.

Fig. 5.19 Hamstring stretch

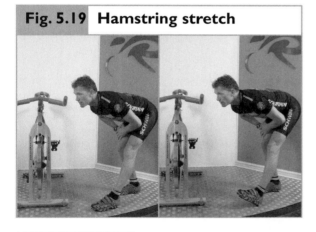

Adductors longus

Find a space and place your feet a little past hip
width apart. Tighten your backside to feel a
slight stretch in the inner thighs (adductors).
Then turn one foot out and drop the knee of the
same side to extend the stretch in the adductor
of the rear leg (see Fig. 5.20).

Fig. 5.20 Adductor stretch

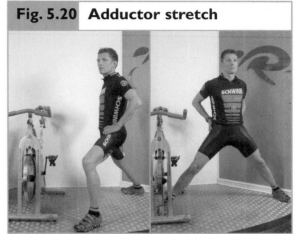

Hip flexor/iliopsoas

From the same position as the previous stretch
gently turn the hips over bringing the ball of the
foot up on the rear leg. Push the hips forwards
and drop the knee of the front foot. Ensure the
knee doesn't go in front of the toes and stays
over the heel (see Fig. 5.21).

For further passive and PNF stretches see
Chapter 7 under 'Training away from the bike'.

Fig. 5.21 Hip flexor stretch

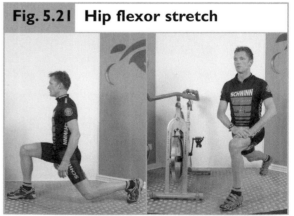

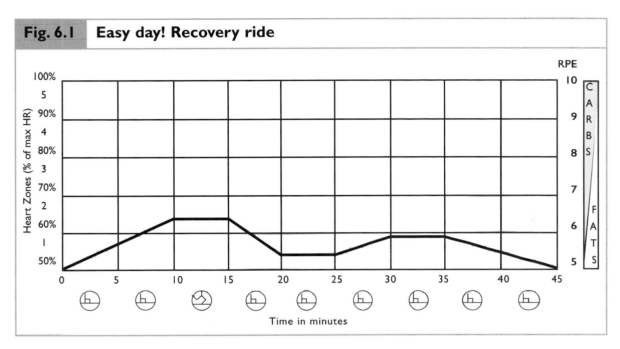

Fig. 6.1 **Easy day! Recovery ride**

Time in minutes

Class profiles

Recovery ride (Fig. 6.1)

This ride can be used for complete beginners, special populations and as an active recovery exercise after intense classes on the schedule or from other training. The heart rate stays below 65% of maximum and hovers between 50 and 65%, between floor of Zone 1 and mid-point of Zone 2. It will be a seated flat technique for most of the class, possibly adding standing flat if the class is advanced and the heart rate can stay low enough.

It could be an ideal class to go over techniques and biomechanics and refine bike position. Music choice will play an important role to keep the class focused.

Rolling roads of England (Fig. 6.2)

This class could be called the 'health benefits' class as it will improve fat metabolism, gain muscle mass and give a good endurance base. Usually ride with heart rates in Zone 2 and 3, 65–75%. If class members are new or struggling, this is a good class for them. It is ideal for selling a concept and educating them while they are on a high from the nature of the class and feeling comfortable, confident and exhilarated. Below 70% the breathing will be comfortable. Above 70% there will be an improvement in the size of blood vessels and in respiratory and cardiac functions; stress-reducing endorphins are released and there is a gradual shift in the fuel utilisation towards carbohydrates. These benefits can last for hours after the class.

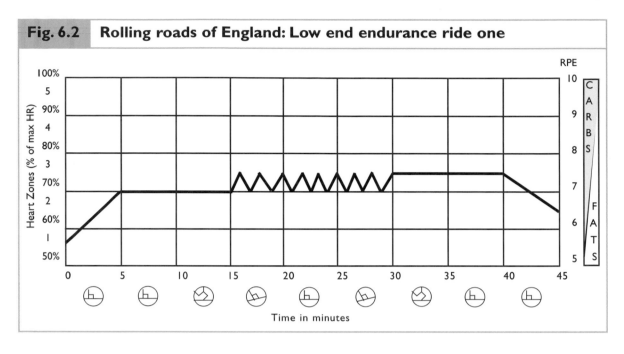

Fig. 6.2   Rolling roads of England: Low end endurance ride one

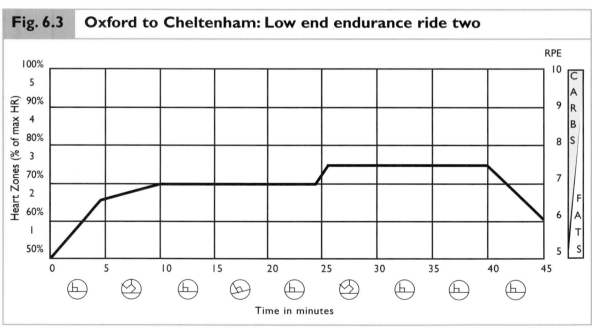

Fig. 6.3   Oxford to Cheltenham: Low end endurance ride two

Fig. 6.4 **London to Birmingham: Low end endurance ride three**

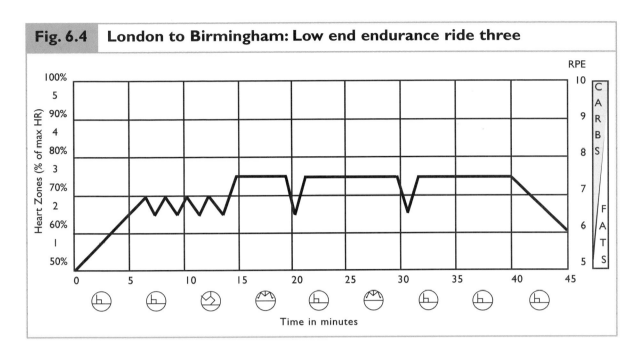

Fig. 6.5 **London to Brighton bike ride: Low end endurance ride four**

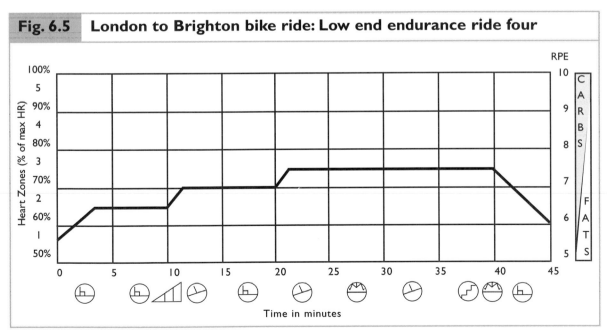

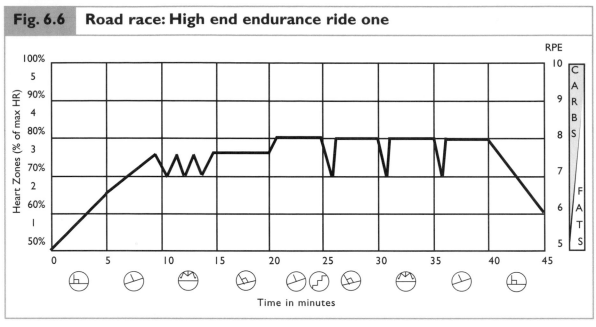

Fig. 6.6   Road race: High end endurance ride one

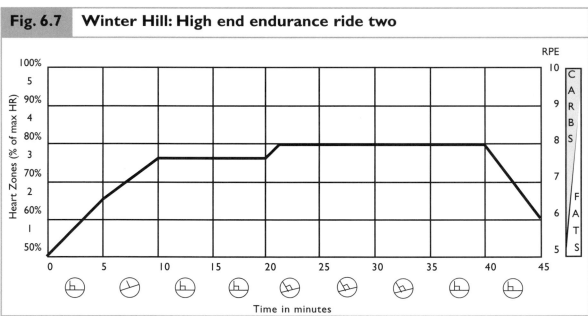

Fig. 6.7   Winter Hill: High end endurance ride two

High end endurance

High end endurance classes are normally 75–85% of maximum; there are huge cardiovascular benefits. You will get the biggest

fitness benefits in the least amount of time. Your body is consuming lots of oxygen and releasing brain chemicals called endorphins that dull pain. Up to the ceiling of Zone 3, 80%, you build up resistance to pain and fatigue. Above

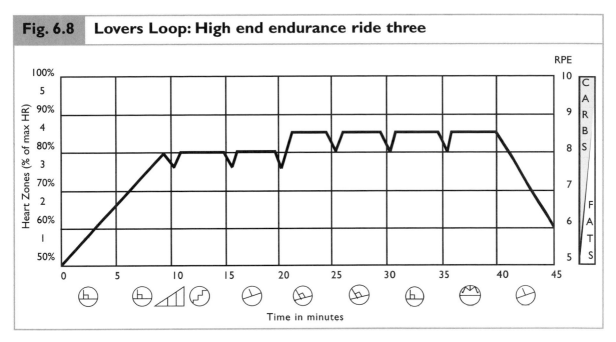

Fig. 6.8 | **Lovers Loop: High end endurance ride three**

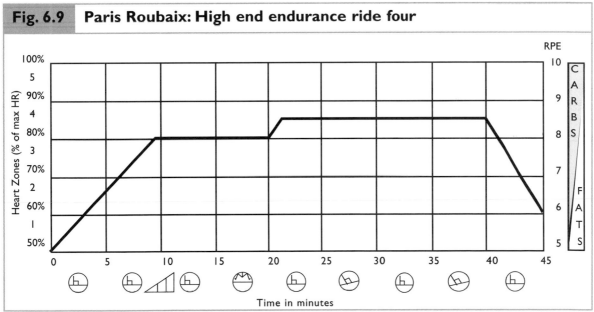

Fig. 6.9 | **Paris Roubaix: High end endurance ride four**

this to the mid-point of Zone 4, 85%, you get fitter and faster, and increase the tolerance to lactic acid production. Breathing is more difficult, and you wouldn't want to hold a conversation. Normally most people's threshold will be around 85%; this will be too stressful for a beginner (see Fig. 6.6–6.9).

Music bpm will play a valuable role as a

guideline to leg speeds (rpm) and become important for safety, focus and motivation. You can add more varied and challenging main sets, including combination flats and hills, and hill climbs (seated and standing).

Competition class

Watch out! These classes are hard work – but fun. Treat them like a race and examine the varying techniques. By the time students are ready to do this class they will be getting fit, so

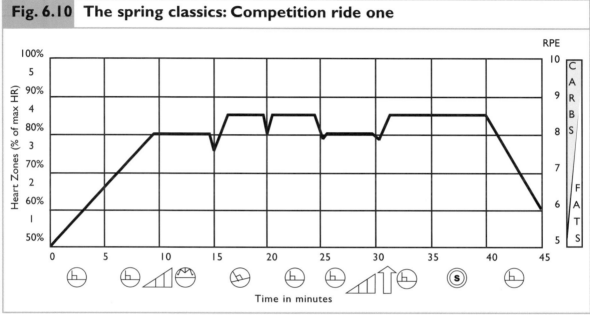

Fig. 6.10 **The spring classics: Competition ride one**

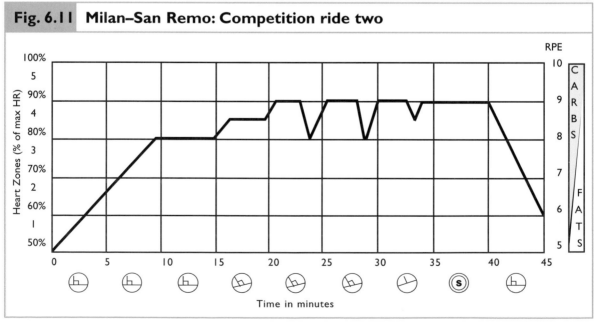

Fig. 6.11 **Milan–San Remo: Competition ride two**

go for it, you can push the class members (remember, they must drink on the move). Focus on moving smoothly through the signs. Recovery can be getting on a wheel (drafting). Be creative, pick music to match the emotions and adrenaline of a race – fast and furious. Use the heart rate guidelines: 80%+ of maximum for the whole class. If you can't visualise this, sit and watch a bike race on television; look for the tactics, the teamwork and the leaders. This will give you good ideas for profiles and techniques as well as terminology (see Fig. 6.10–Fig. 6.13).

Fig. 6.12 The criterium: Competition ride three

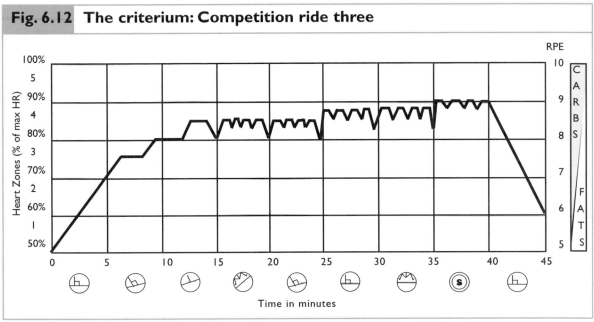

Fig. 6.13 Final stage: Tour de France: Competition ride four

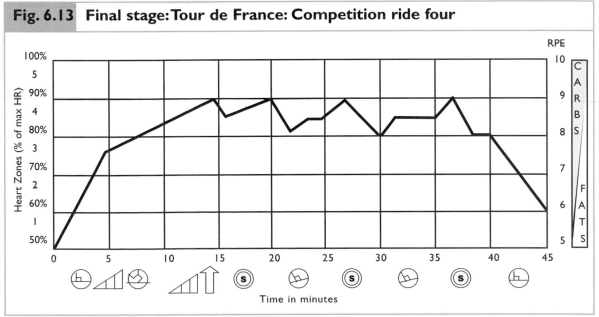

Criterium class

This ride is a favourite of the regulars! A ride of five laps – or more, it is up to you. Although we have shown a different technique for each lap, you can make every lap the same using a number of techniques, e.g. One 5-minute lap = seated flat 1 minute, seated climb 50 seconds, standing flat 40 seconds (shout 'half way!'), combination flat 1 minute, seated climb towards the finish 1 minute, seated flat for the last 30 seconds through the finish tunnel. On the last lap there is obviously a sprint of 15 seconds for the line. Winner takes all! During the ride you keep everyone in line and on the wheels, observing the correct pedalling guidelines for each technique.

Tour de France

Visit the French capital and race around the famous monument on the final day of the Tour de France, the biggest and most famous bike race in the world. This is a super-advanced race class. Plenty of controlled 15-second sprints with hills and pace changes. Not for the faint-hearted or riders of only average fitness. You have to train for this one. Heart rates are high and a recovery ride or day off the next day is required!

Hill classes (Fig. 6.14–6.17)

The hill rides can be just as challenging and just as rewarding as the competition classes. You feel as if you have really accomplished something when you reach the top and it is all downhill to home.

The rpms are 60–80 bpm, and so the tempo and beat of the music changes. Don't forget the air in the highest mountains is damp and thin – use visualisation carefully to create an awesome ride.

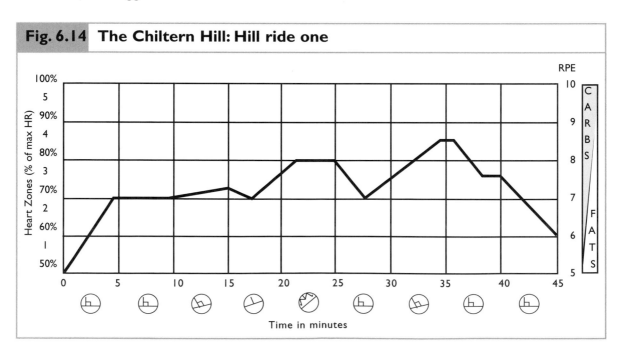

Fig. 6.14 **The Chiltern Hill: Hill ride one**

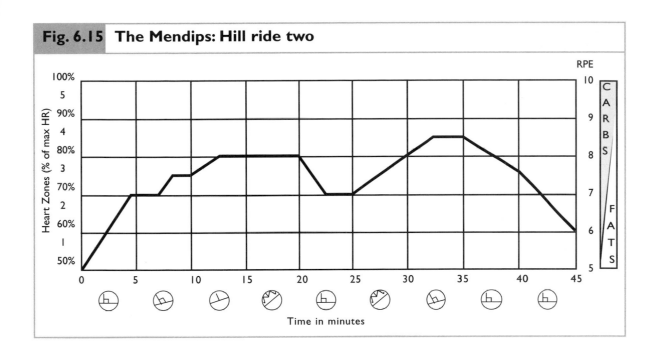

Fig. 6.15 The Mendips: Hill ride two

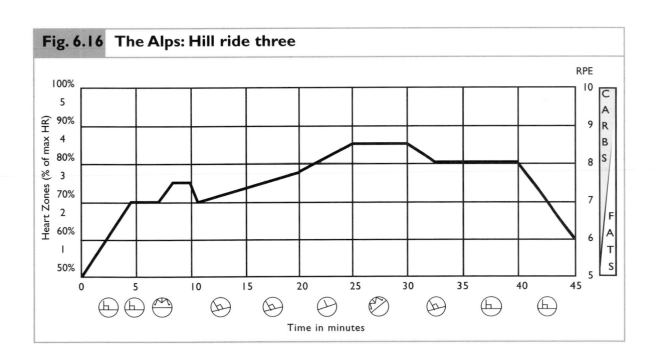

Fig. 6.16 The Alps: Hill ride three

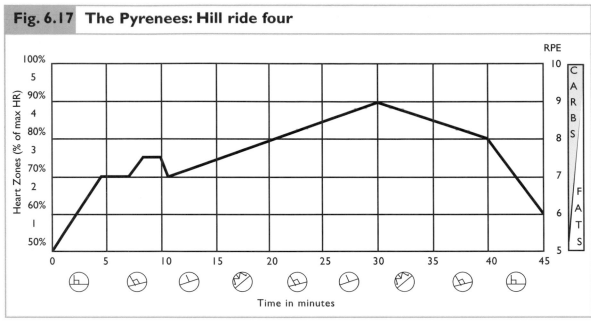

Fig. 6.17 The Pyrenees: Hill ride four

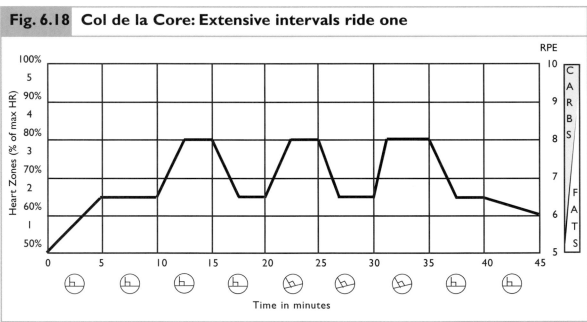

Fig. 6.18 Col de la Core: Extensive intervals ride one

Extensive intervals

The extensive interval classes are challenging within the heart rate guidelines 65–85% of max heart rate. However, you don't have to go to the highest percentages but can remain within 65–75% or 70–80% for your intervals. At the top end these will increase anaerobic threshold, VO2max and lactate tolerance. You stay within

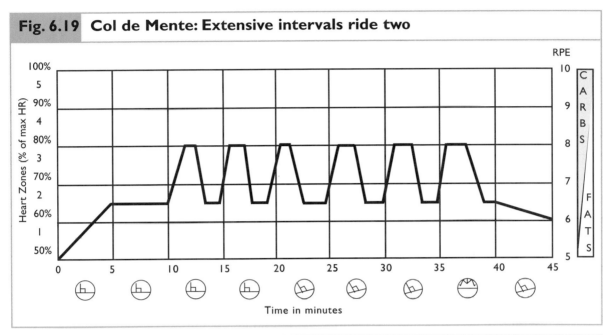

Fig. 6.19 Col de Mente: Extensive intervals ride two

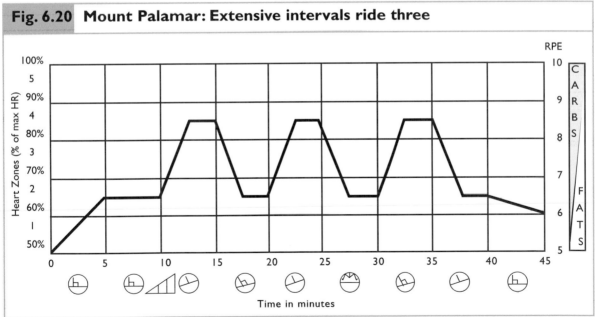

Fig. 6.20 Mount Palamar: Extensive intervals ride three

the threshold, so you will be burning oxygen and some fat. Use the phrases in the music to build in the intervals. Recovery time is equal to interval time.

Try to change the music style for this type of class and the intensive interval class, you should use all the variables to keep them working and motivated.

97

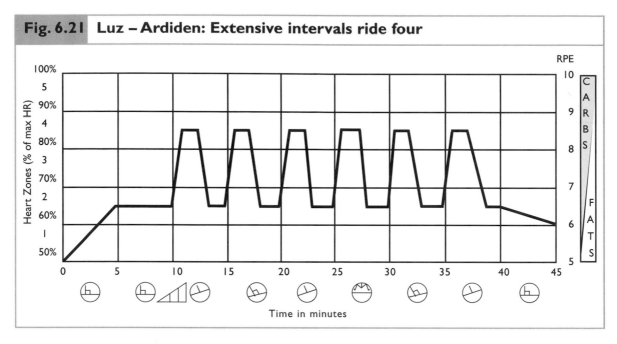

Fig. 6.21 Luz – Ardiden: Extensive intervals ride four

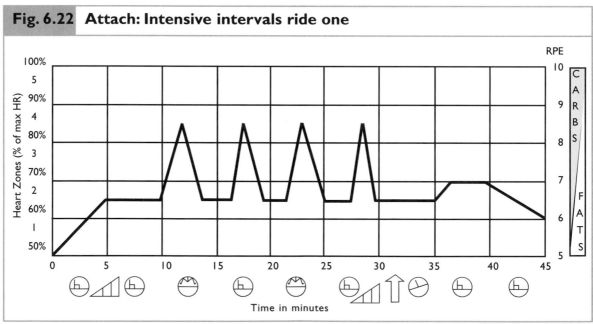

Fig. 6.22 Attach: Intensive intervals ride one

Intensive intervals

Intensive intervals will take the class above the anaerobic threshold 65–90% of max, so the intervals will be short and the recovery time will be twice as long. You will be working with challenging music and within the technique

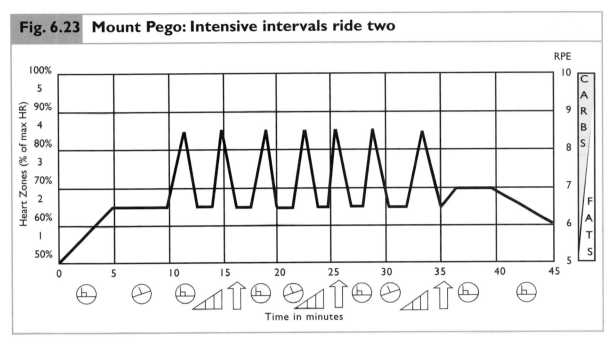

Fig. 6.23 Mount Pego: Intensive intervals ride two

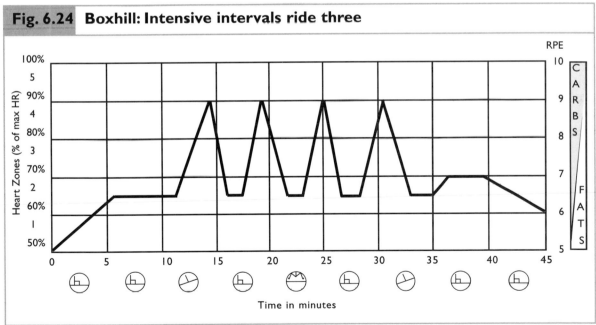

Fig. 6.24 Boxhill: Intensive intervals ride three

guidelines. These are advanced classes if you take the interval to the highest percentage. There is hypertrophy of the heart, increases in VO2 max and improvements in the ability to tolerate lactic acid.

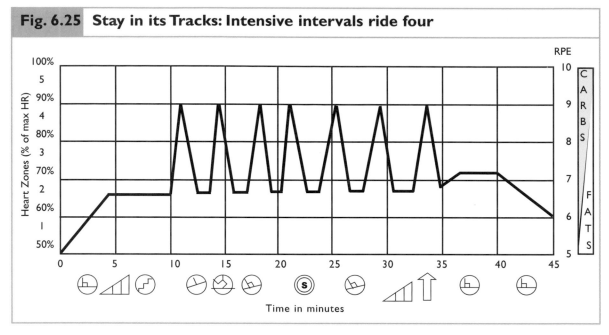

Fig. 6.25 Stay in its Tracks: Intensive intervals ride four

Studio-cycling instructor grid

Table 6.1 covers most of the points that will help you to prepare for teaching a successful studio-cycling class in a club.

Ten goals for new studio-cycling instructors

- Ride the bikes as much as possible for your own practice and to get comfortable so that you can lead by example. You don't have to be the fittest person in the class but you must be able to lead the class on the bikes.
- Practise with other instructors before you teach your first class and set up some trial classes with your friends, ask for their feedback. However, don't leave it too long otherwise your confidence and enthusiasm may diminish.
- Put yourself on a progressive studio-cycling training programme, so that you can go through what the class members will. You can then teach and coach from experience.
- Recognise your clients, find out about them, why they are training and what their background is, then you can set up a training programme to meet their needs.
- Use the easy-to-use studio-cycling maps and select music that matches the signs.
- Create your own progressive profile maps as your classes develop.
- Keep a full record/logbook of your class maps and training schedule so you can see what worked and what could have been better.
- Attend other instructors' classes, discuss and critique each other. Constructive criticism will help you to become the best studio-cycling instructor possible.
- If you don't know something, research it, find out and understand it so that you can give an informed answer to the class member.
- Keep an open mind!

Table 6.1	**Essential teaching points for instructors**
PREPARATION	**Basic understanding of all aspects of health and fitness.** A core knowledge of basic anatomy and physiology as well as progression training and of course flexibility and energy systems.
	Accredited qualification to teach studio cycling. You must attend the relevant studio-cycling courses and pass all the necessary exams, thereafter refreshing periodically with continuing education in levels of studio cycling.
	Full understanding of what you are teaching. There is no better way to teach or coach than from experience and by example. Try the programmes yourself, teach classes, and then attend other classes with other instructors. You will then understand what your class members are experiencing.
	Work on your weaknesses and practise. If you don't know your weaknesses get feedback from other instructors who teach your classes. Monitor your techniques in a mirror, practise and refine them.
	Class size (number of bikes) and room logistics. How many bikes can you fit in the space you have, and what formation will you put them in to get the best out of the class. Be imaginative with your designs, still allowing perfect vision both ways: from you to the class member and from them to you. Provide plenty of space between the bikes for access and to stop heart monitor crosstalk.
	Studio coordinator or your club contact. If you cover classes, who is your contact? Establish a good rapport with them so that they help you and understand your requirements before, during and after the class. Always have the names of the relevant people who can help you with maintenance and problem-solving, cleaning materials, lubricants, etc.
	Arrive with enough set-up time and be available to greet clients. Try to make sure you are the first person there. There is nothing more unprofessional than an instructor turning up when everyone is already on the bikes, especially if it's a beginners' class. In the latter case they must not be on the bikes unless you are there, so there is a definite safety issue. If you are delayed you must inform the club so that they can arrange for someone to be there until you arrive.
	Number of clients – name sheet. Know the names of your class members – they know yours! It is unprofessional not to remember their names. When they tell you for the first time, keep repeating it in your head over and over again. Say it out aloud to them before you move on. You should have a list of participants who have booked for your class; add another column to it dated the following week, and when you take the register or payment (if applicable) ask each member there and then if they are coming. If they say 'yes', they are less likely to let you down the next time. It is like a contract. They will feel obliged to contact you if they cannot make it. It avoids occasions when someone fails to show and leaves a bike free that someone else would have liked to have.

CD player/changer. Does the club have a CD player, or do you only have tapes? If CDs, how many will you use, and are you planning to change them during the class? If you get sweat on them when you make the change they will skip just when you are in the middle of a vital sequence and this will spoil important continuity, focus and motivation.

Suitable safe area – space the bikes. Is the area safe to put the bikes in, leaving walkways free and adequate entry and exit points?

Shoes, bike shorts, jersey, towel and water bottle (filled with water or energy drink). Does everyone have suitable footwear, have you informed them of the benefits of rigid bike shoes with cleats. Bike shorts which have a special pad in are much more comfortable as they have been anatomically designed and treated with antibacterial materials. The clothing material will be important for comfort as it will wick away moisture and sweat and feel more comfortable. Everyone must have towel and water – towels to wipe off the sweat and water to hydrate the body. Tests have shown that when people come straight to the class from work around 90% will be a little dehydrated. Drink before, during and after the class – see and feel the difference !

Music prepared and selected to match the class profile. All your music will match the theme and rhythms you require for terrains and rpms. Count the bpm so you can advise the class if they can follow or set their own rpms. Use variety, and understand you can ride different terrains to any piece of music. Don't use the same music every class.

Water and spare bottles for class members who forget theirs. Know that at least one or more people will forget their water bottle. Have some spares filled and ready by your bike just in case. No one is expected or allowed to ride a 45-minute class without access to water.

Spray and paper towels. The bikes must be kept clean. The first rule is to provide spray and paper towels. The class members are told at the end of every class to clean their own bikes down. Their efforts will probably not be good enough and instructors need to check every bike after each class. Dirty or sweaty bikes must be cleaned before the next class. No one should be expected to ride in another person's sweat.

Emergency exits, first aid and safety procedures for the club you teach in. Ensure that everyone knows the procedure in case of emergency evacuation, who the safety officer is and where the first aid kit and fire extinguishers are.

Arrive early (see above)

Time with your clients
- **Approachability.** Spend time talking, smiling, looking around before class.
- **Name.** Play the name game –see above.
- **History.** Why are they in your class, what training have they done in the past and recently?
- **Goals.** Have they set any short, medium or long term goals. You can help them decide if they are realistic.

Confidence in yourself. The more you practise, the more confidence you will have. Practice makes perfect.

PROFESSIONALISM

Attitude, appearance, kit, change of kit if needed. Dry, sweet-smelling and clean! New, no holes, and part of the club uniform if possible. Clean-shaven, healthy and smart.

Present a healthy, active and smart image, i.e. fitness and eating habits. Don't chew gum in the class, try to eat healthily in front of people. Always try to show that you care about what you put into your body. If you are going to eat chocolate bars do so off-site. Project a clean-living, healthy image at all times.

Show you care. When you arrive talk *to* people not *at* them, be concerned, and listen to their problems.

Be positive and personable. Look bright and happy, ask questions and respond by laughing and tell interesting stories and jokes.

Talk to the club management – number of class members, equipment quality control. Ensure you know how many people are coming to your class, and that all the equipment is clean and in working order, including the music, PA and microphone.

Self-evaluation and class report. Ask the class if they enjoyed it, speak to one person who you know well and doesn't mind giving you negative feedback if they have to. If you teach a master class or a beginners' class you can hand out an evaluation sheet with key questions that are going to help you improve.

Feedback from staff, management and class members. Talk to everyone after the class, or the week later once the euphoria has died down.

Benefits to your business. By being as professional as you can you will gain respect, have full classes and recruit personal training classes.

Promoting HRMs, shoes, shorts and other associated products that aid a good class. To understand and realise the benefits of quality equipment and products and promote them ethically to the class.

CONTENT

Class register. A list of all class members checked before class as they arrive.

Class plan. Prepare a class plan with frequency, intensity, time, technique and music.

Techniques. Correct technique of class members and demonstrations by instructor.

Practical tests etc. Tests to measure heart rate response and muscle balances.

RPE. Rate of perceived exertion scale 1–10.

Heart zones. Dosage of each of the five zones for multiple benefits.

Music. Choice of rhythms and beats per minute to match class profiles.

Focus and concentration. Mental training to improve focus of class members through breathing techniques, music, intervals, biomechanics and goal-setting.

DELIVERY

Timing in relation to auditory and visual delivery. Verbally give the technique then allow time to practise and work with it. Demonstrate the technique then encourage the class to follow.

Style and creativity. Be imaginative and descriptive.

Motivation. Use the techniques and understand how they can motivate groups and individuals.

- **Don't be autocratic.** Most of the time it is better not to shout at the class but rather use skills and techniques that will improve class and individual response.
- **Enthusiasm.** Show the correct levels of enthusiasm to motivate the class.
- **Coach.** Understand the differences between the requirements of a coach and an instructor.
- **Discipline.** Use control to keep discipline within the class and the individuals who need it.

Timings. When to deliver a command or technique. **Promptness** – always be there 15 minutes before the class, and finish the class when it it advertised in case people are using the class like a clock. **Plan** the classes so that they have elements of progression in intensity and duration. **Set time** – know how long each part of the class will take so that you can show the class at the beginning, set the time so that each part fits perfectly into a full class.

Intuition of clients – observe clients and make sure their technique is correct. Where there's confusion show alternative explanation or analogy. Questions involve the whole group – avoid one or two people answering all the questions.

Material progresses logically and clearly at a pace with students' learning ability. Don't give the class techniques it cannot cope with.

Review. Go over old technique/biomechanics or sets with intervals that have been completed and goals that have been achieved.

Link areas to each other. Seamless music changes, techniques that flow into each other, intervals that inspire and motivate.

Divert questions that aren't relevant, i.e. positive reinforcement (smile), 'Yes, we'll come on to that in a minute'. Make sure you do. But focus on the control needed and important techniques.

Receptiveness of what you are teaching — i.e. are they tired? Empathy to how they feel because you are feeling it too.

Intuition and ability to change. Do members need a water/towel break etc? Are they enjoying it? You may need to change your style.

Confidence and knowledge. Show your skills when you need to, be calm, be emotive, be enthusiastic, be in control, show you know exactly what you are doing.

Explain difficult areas clearly. Practise with clear and audible descriptions, watch for understanding and key changes in.

Good delivery comes with experience. You can't be the best without skills and experience but the best will come to you if you keep learning, practise and accept criticism. Be humble and open-minded. There is always a better way!

Be available to clients prior to class. Make sure you have plenty of time to set up and pack up before and after a class so that you can interact with the class members who will want your opinions and information on training, diet and other things that you may not feel are important but will make the world of difference to that person.

INTERACTION/COMMUNICATION

What you say and do. Everyone will copy you so make sure to give sound advice and instructions as well as show perfect technique all the time; lead by example.

Eye contact. Look at people before the class, don't avoid eye contact.

Your ability and confidence will communicate skills that you don't even know you have.

Recapping at the end of each technique and of the class. Ensure the class and individuals understand and comprehend how to execute each technique and why they are doing it. Part of this education process will be to go through the profiles and techniques that were used in the class.

Identifying members experiencing difficulty and offer support. A coach's eye can only be developed if the right skills and understanding have been taught and practised repeatedly.

Prompt answers. If you are asked a question, give a good simple answer; if you don't know the answer you must find out as soon as possible. Nobody expects you to know everything.

Examples of experience. By showing the experience and knowledge with positive examples and successes you can win over even the most negative of people.

Observation. Explain what you have seen and how it can be improved or changed.

Questions. Pass on any questions you can't answer to your teacher or management.

Feedback objectives. Give feedbacks on what it is you are trying to achieve and if they are being met.

Feedback types: visual, verbal or auditory, heart rate, kinaesthetic types.

Time to talk. Provide time for members to talk at end of class.

Contact with key personnel. Stay in contact with the club coordinators, management.

ASSESSMENT

Ability during class. Are the objectives being met, do the class members know the techniques

Confidence. Are you confident in front of the class and are the class members confident to attempt the techniques or challenges?

Control. Do you have control of the class at all times, before, during and after the class?

Safety. Are your techniques and challenges safe, are the stretches safe or perhaps contra-indicated?

Clients' evaluation of your class: verbal, or on class evaluation form provided by club.

Launching and promoting studio cycling

Marketing and promotion

- ⚷ Experience has shown that marketing and promotion are vital to your own classes as well as the success of the club. This is not because we have a weak concept but because people see studio cycling in different ways.
- ⚷ First impressions are important, and because classes look tough, with everyone sweating, it can give the impression of elitism or that a high level of fitness is required just to take part. This is where you can help by talking to people. Word of mouth is your best weapon as long as what is being said is positive.
- ⚷ Encourage people to experience the unique feel and easiness of pedalling. Explain the principle of riding to the rhythm of music.
- ⚷ Encourage all frontline staff such as receptionists, secretaries, membership sales people, gym instructors, personal trainers, duty managers, restaurant/bar staff, whether they are full- or part-time, to attend classes, so that they can enthuse about studio cycling so as to sell the idea and create a buzz about it.
- ⚷ Studio cycling is ideally suited to retain existing members, re-enthuse old past members and entice new ones. It is a new service that can be used to spearhead club membership drives.
- ⚷ New members should be given studio-cycling inductions when they join, along with other things such as fitness assessments, etc.
- ⚷ Studio cycling is not aerobics, there is no technical coordination needed, therefore you can identify a whole new type of potential member, who can enjoy class exercise training for the first time.
- ⚷ The bikes are easy to move on their wheels; use this feature to hold classes in high-profile positions such as the bar area, reception area or gym. This will create awareness; there will be no one who has not heard or seen a studio-cycling class.
- ⚷ Link up with local businesses such as the local bike shop and perhaps offer staff discounts for referrals. Contact local bike clubs to offer classes during the winter.
- ⚷ The best start when you launch studio cycling in your club will come after a little extra time and effort.
- ⚷ Design a press release, perhaps through your marketing department, although we have found better results occur if several qualified instructors have a brain-storming session and the best bits are taken from each person's ideas. Add them together and you will have a great press release to go in a club newsletter or to the local newspapers along with an invitation to a special class for press and VIPs at the launch party.

Write your own press release:

_____
_____
_____
_____
_____
_____

The launch

By now, everything has been done to ensure maximum publicity. Don't start teaching too soon, try to practise behind closed doors with friends, staff or other instructors. Remember you are working to your own training plan, to get fit enough to lead by example or just confident enough to lead the class along the set journey practised. This is the time to publicise the launch date; why not have a count-down – ten, nine days to go, right down to 'The Day'.

🚲 Set the launch date. Make sure the class is full, even oversubscribed; make it hard to get into the class so that you create the feeling of high worth. You must work hard to ensure every class for the first month is FULL! Have reserve lists; if there's a drop-out call the reserves. Still one place left? Draft someone in, another instructor will do.

🚲 Invite a local celebrity to open or ride in the first class.

Innovations

The class environment of studio cycling allows it to be imaginative. In fact the classes are limited only to the power of your imagination. You have a captive audience at your disposal – use it! The feedback you are given will let you know if members are responding to your ideas.

Tried and tested class ideas

🚲 The progressive training approach will let your clients know that you are looking after their training programmes for them. Within these classes you can incorporate all the basic training levels and principles.

🚲 Themed classes – there are too many theme ideas to list, just use your imagination. We have done Christmas studio cycling with Santa, wearing fancy dress; candlelit classes for the spiritual spins; charity classes raising money; team-building classes; rugby and football team classes; visualised races. I am sure you will think of many more, perhaps even better ones.

> **Instructor tip:**
>
> Keep your classes simple!

Advanced studio-cycling techniques for existing instructors

You may feel after a while that you have reached a plateau and don't seem to be improving; the only way forwards is to go back to basics. Strengthen your foundations so that you can build and grow further. This next phase of training is very simple, perhaps easier than the initial phase of learning how to be a studio-cycling instructor. It allows you to implement all the elements that you have been teaching; however, now that you have the core knowledge you can increase your understanding where, when and why you should use these elements. Understanding what you already know is the key.

Perhaps one of the most important parts of teaching studio-cycling classes is having a structure to your class. If you feel that you have not practised this from the onset now is the time to start changing your ways. Your class structure may not always go to plan; this is normal. As an instructor you know that you must adapt the programme to suit the level of the individual. You are now an advanced studio-cycling instructor, this is the time to start building the techniques together, playing with rhythms, heart rates, goals and the mind.

Advanced heart rate monitoring during a studio-cycling class

As an advanced instructor you should now know a considerable amount about your body and particularly how your heart rate responds to exercise with the demands of teaching and training.

It is by using a heart rate monitor and seeing for yourself how your heart rate responds that you are able to gain experience and knowledge that you can pass on the benefits to class members. You may find that some of your class members still do not possess a heart rate monitor, in which case it may be wise to advise them that your classes will be heart-rate related and that they can purchase heart rate monitors cheaply in any good sports shops. Alternatively, why not provide some monitors for the class members to use? Here is a chance to get the station bag out and hand out monitors to all those who don't have one. If you *are* teaching heart rate, always make sure that you are wearing a monitor yourself; remember, you are the one that sets the example.

The errors of manual pulse-taking

Many people try to monitor their heart rate by stopping their activity to take a pulse. This is not the best idea, because where do you start and stop counting?

- If you are just one or two beats off in a 6-second count, that is a difference of 10–20 beats. Also, when you stop to take your pulse, your heart rate decreases rapidly.
- In 6 seconds the rate may drop by 15–30 beats or more.
- Interestingly, the light pressure used to take your pulse from the carotid artery in the neck can trigger a rapid slowing of heart rate.

Studio-cycling training programme protocol

Have you ever thought about what training you did last week or how you felt, but you can't quite remember? If the answer is yes, then the answer is simple – keep a logbook. Professional athletes keep a logbook of their training, their achievable goals, illness, injury, lack of motivation or tiredness. As a studio-cycling instructor you should do the same; by honestly

logging what training you have done you are able to identify at a glance whether you are becoming ill or overtraining, or even if you are improving your fitness or strength. In the initial chapters we recommended you keep a log of your class profiles. Even better – keep a log of all your training.

Coaching oneself is an incredibly hard thing to do; human nature tends to convince you to reason against balance. If you coach yourself you may find that you want to do more than is necessary and not allow proper recovery after hard or long training. This doesn't happen with another person coaching you because he or she will be more objective. A good coach will recognise how much training is best, when to increase it and when to back off, and can motivate a student who doesn't do enough training. In Chapter 4 there are tests to use; to a certain extent they can be used to coach yourself, although the inexperienced might find it quite daunting. Even the most experienced athlete has trouble writing the best schedules.

Training rules: duration and progression

Improvements result from *cause and adaptation*, i.e. for the body to grow and improve it must be overloaded, break down, and be allowed to recover so that it grows back more efficient, bigger, faster etc.

With studio cycling the *normal limits don't apply* because the exercise is non-impact; it uses an excellent warm-up and recovery, allowing for muscular warming, while the heart rate is kept lower than normal. Then, through gradual increase of intensities, the main set can be harder than normal, but with the muscles still hot the intensity is lowered during the cool-down, which in turn aids *super recovery*.

One week of the schedule is micro-cycle, one month a meso-cycle, and a twelve-week period is a macro-cycle.

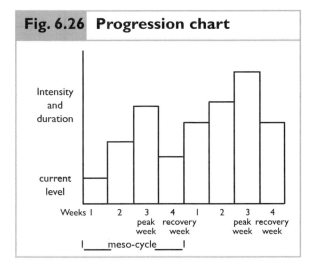

Fig. 6.26 Progression chart

It may help to write out your own new goals along with your own month's training plan.

- Short term………..
- Medium term……..
- Long term…………

Teaching off the bike

Teaching off the bike allows you to take command of your members individually. It can increase their motivation and build personal commitment.

An instructor should only get off the bike in order to:

- Assist a client with their position or look for potential poor bike set-up.
- Review a client's cycling technique.
- Give individual motivation or improve technique.

As the instructor you should always lead by example. It is vital that you pace yourself during the class – you should never get off the bike and teach. If you need to do this you should not yet be teaching; instead practise

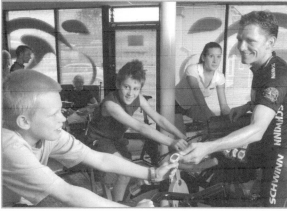

Fig. 6.27 Teaching off the bike with juniors

with friends and colleagues before you start your own classes.

The way you dismount at the end of the class is very important; the class will be watching the instructor. If you were to jump off the bike without touching the brake there is a likelihood that some of the members may do the same.

Advanced cycling techniques

The following cycling techniques can be used in your classes; whilst they are not vital to a class they are used to balance leg strength, redress specific weakness and promote core balance. They are often used by cyclists as a rehabilitation technique or simply to build strength.

- **One leg spinning** – if you are unsure of the ability of the class you should not teach this technique, as it can be dangerous. The rider must carefully take one foot out of the toe clip. Use time or counting to set session goals (see Fig. 6.28). (Do not use this exercise as part of the main set, it is designed only to discover if you have a weaker leg.)
- **Increasing speed during a climb** – keep resistance set high and get the class to follow your lead by increasing rpms.

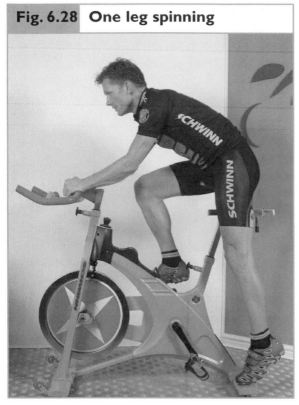

Fig. 6.28 One leg spinning

- **Focusing on specific muscles** – identify a muscle or area of the body and explore its 'feel'. Use this technique to focus on a weaker leg.

Fig. 6.29 Example of poor posture

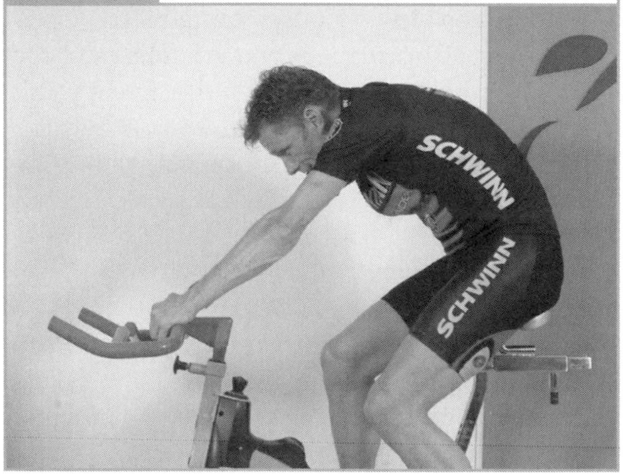

- **Lower back neutral position** – try to allow the back to stay in a relaxed position without being strained. Set goals of lowering the handlebars and/or moving the saddle back. Incorporate hip flexibility and lower back exercises.
- **Deep head, neck, shoulder relaxation techniques** – focus on relaxing individual muscles; use breathing technique while listing body parts. Work from the head to the toes.

Advanced training

- **Intervals: to fatigue** – set the goal, i.e. time and total number of intervals for class members depending on level of ability.
- **Intervals adding resistance** – as above but gradually add resistance.
- **Intervals increasing speed** – set a start and finish cadence or rpm or simply allow people to feel the resistance. Use this as a power set within a main set – very advanced.
- **Timing your efforts and measuring recovery** – use a heart rate drop from a set maximum (remember not everyone will have the same maximum heart rate) and always use the same recovery time to measure progress. Change the types of tests to challenge the class within the 45 minutes.
- **Resistance cadence counting** – add resistance and increase your revolutions up to 5-second max spin; with the toe clips loose take your feet carefully out of the pedals and count how many times the cranks rotate. Now you can ask the class to set the resistance to a desired level, and have them all ride at their own level. It can be any number of rotations; a good start is five. This is a short test and needs to be controlled. Show the class exactly how to do it first. It is an excellent test to show people how little resistance there is on their flywheel.

- **One arm climb** – hand position: standing climb only, high resistance for safety and control. Feel the specific quad muscles work to increase lateral balance and individual leg strength. This will teach the individuals the benefits of muscle balancing and whether their leg strength needs work.

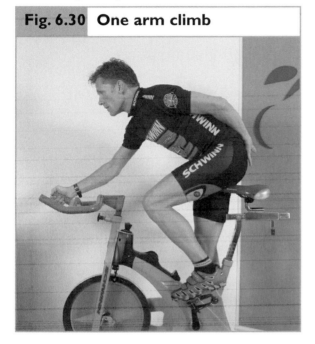

Fig. 6.30 **One arm climb**

Advanced focusing (for the mind and body)

This powerful tool allows the class to block out external distractions and work with their 'Energy'. We have previously discussed the importance of focusing and visualisation and will continue to do so as your class learns and grows with you, the instructor. You must understand why you use a technique to make it advanced.

Tools for focusing are:

- Breathing – rhythmic breathing at predetermined speeds can aid focus.
- Music – will help block out distractions such as pain, light, movements etc.

- The instructor can use key verbal or non-verbal commands and suggestions to increase individual focus.
- Fixed objects – try and teach the class to focus on a fixed object for an extended period of time; this will take the mind off the physical distraction and aid concentration on the set task.
- The student's own body – when focusing on a part of the body the class isolates thoughts to that area. By exploring the body part's movement, feeling its effort and relaxing or working it harder, they are now able to focus.
- Counting for a period of time will allow the mind to focus on relaxing during effort.
- Time can be used to focus on targets and goals. Satisfaction can be gained by reaching the target. For how long can they ride in one position or resistance?
- Sight – when opening or closing your eyes you will cut out or close off distractions; if necessary, build in distraction workloads to aid progressive focusing.

Focusing the mind and body is vital for development, and is a tool that allows the individual to progress to higher levels.

Advanced verbal suggestions

Here are some key verbal suggestions that the instructor can use. Have you already been using them? Do you know why? That is how this technique becomes advanced – if you know why!

- Relax your upper body.
- Close your eyes.
- Breathe.
- Nothing worth doing is ever easy.
- Find the energy inside.
- You feel strong.
- It feels good, stay strong etc.
- Go for it!

Verbal suggestions should all be positive!

Non-verbal suggestions
- Eye contact.
- Exaggerated body movements.
- Strong techniques.
- Teaching off the bike.
- Using heart rate monitoring.
- Visualization.
- Mirroring.

Team building

Start with a partner, and set your bikes opposite one another. You are your partner and they are you – a mirror image. One person starts a technique and their partner has to mirror it. If the partner wants to change the technique they can; the first person must follow until they too change the technique, and so it goes on. Only allow simple techniques and use emotive music. This can be useful towards the end of a hard class if you want to maintain pressure for one more set.

Advanced goal setting

Advanced motivation can come from goal setting. Set personal goals for each class member. You can use goals such as working on technique deficiencies or weaknesses with mental and physical efforts. The work you do with an individual could be longer, intense efforts – but think about the individual and what makes them tick, what inspires them; this will come from interaction and observation. As their coach, this is your job.

You will find 'advanced goal setting' is reaching the goal and changing it.

Example:
- Combination flats and hills/jumping: Class level is 100 jumps per class – when you reach 100, agree with the class to do ten or twenty more. You have made a contract with the class and they have achieved more than they thought they would do.
- Hill climb classes: During each hill, class clients climb for a fixed period of time plus the extra goal you set them. Get to the top and ask them to climb more. This is advanced goal setting!

Advanced visualisation

- 'You can see the end of the road'.
- 'At the end of the road you can stop'.
- 'When you get to the top, it is all downhill!'.

These are all examples of visualisation that you may have used; giving motivation through visualisation is not new. Now you have to become creative and clever. Your clients will be used to this form of goading and cajoling. You must make them want to get to the top or to the end of that road first. But not just by making it so tough that they are desperate to finish – that is easy. Think now how you can achieve advanced visualisation.

The answer is not easy, however we can use guidelines:
- Positive attitude.
- Self-awareness.
- New senses with new challenges.
- Change the goal and image.

By now you should have a fair few ideas on which to expand your knowledge. Studio cycling is not regimented by rules and etiquette, it enables you to experiment. Some of your ideas will work, some won't but you will never know which unless you try! Just keep it safe and simple.

DIFFERENT FORMS OF STUDIO CYCLING 7

Corporate studio cycling

The corporate studio-cycling market can include large or small companies that have their own gyms and studios. Thousands of companies up and down the country have negotiated corporate deals with their local health and fitness clubs proving that health and fitness certainly does have benefits in relieving stress and enabling you to forget about your work routine.

The corporate world is an extremely large and affluent market group for the fitness industry. Much time and effort is spent marketing to this key target group; methods can include offering special group membership discounts, etc. However, perhaps the most important part will be the fitness programmes that the clubs offer to the company employees.

Studio-cycling classes are ideal for companies as they offer individual exercise within groups of people with a common goal. The groups can consist of employees from the same company or department, or even across departments to enhance team-building elements.

First look at the broad spectrum of people who work in companies:

Thin and unfit
Fat and unfit
Thin and fit
Fat and fit.

People are different shapes and sizes, within 16–65-year age groups and of all levels of ability and fitness. There is such a broad range that there will be scope for many different and specific classes:

Think of corporate studio-cycling names:
Rookies/beginners/novice/apprentice class
Intermediate/business class/sport class
Advanced/executive class/competition class.

Corporate gyms potentially cater for more less-fit personnel than do health and fitness clubs, because they are actually reaching a market of people who wouldn't normally go anywhere near a gym. This can be due to the stigma attached to health clubs: 'They are only for the beautiful people, or for posers!' Many people are unwilling because publicity from health clubs shows ideal body shapes, toned and muscular, displayed on posters and flyers. In reality we all know this picture is not true, but nevertheless this can be enough to put people off joining a gym for life! Bring the gym to the company and introduce health and safety recommendations, and there is the potential for these people to find themselves in this new, exciting – but sometimes daunting – environment. It is within this newfound environment that studio cycling can play an important role, if implemented correctly.

Watching a studio-cycling class in action can have a negative effect, as the class members are quite often hot and sweaty, and pedalling fast. Many people look at this and think to themselves that they are not fit enough. Instead, offer inductions into the gym and studio cycling. An instructor will go through the same process as in a normal beginners' class, but one to one. Set up a mini-class with two bikes facing each other (see Fig. 7.1).

During this opportunity it will be important to get across key concepts and benefits:
• Studio cycling is for everyone.

Fig. 7.1 | Two bikes facing

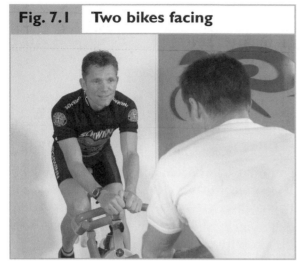

- Safety – flywheel and its advantages.
- Ability to set your own pace and resistance.
- Warm-up benefits that include core temperature (speeding up metabolism).
- Raising threshold and fat burning range.
- Efficient recovery extends time for metabolism due to heat; prevents blood pooling, recycles lactic acid.

Sit on a bike opposite the client and run through a mini-class; the length will be up to you and your client's ability and fitness. Observe the leg-speed guidelines and in some cases reduce these. Heart zones will be a very useful way to ensure he or she is working at a comfortable level with the resistance you ask to be set.

By working one to one with the client you will be able to instil correct technique and focus, which will allow them to get comfortable quickly. This 15–20 minute mini-session will help the client gain the confidence to move on to the beginner/apprentice class within the club timetable.

Heart Zones – 'emotional hearts'

Sally Edwards' corporate programme 'Blitz' focuses not only on heart rate programming but also on the 'emotional heart'. The reasoning behind this is that there are five emotional zones just like the five heart zones. As a person moves through the zones the stress levels change (see Table 7.1).

Table 7.1 | Emotional Heart Zones®

Zone number	Emotional Zone	Zone Description	Zone Benefit
5	Red Zone	Out of control, frantic, total panic, disconnected, emergency	Toxic
4	Distress Zone	Worried, anxious, angry, scattered, fearful, reactive	Cautious Alert
3	Performance Zone	Focused, in the flow, positive stress, fulfilment, completion	Achievements
2	Productive Zone	High concentration, effective, energetic, prolific	Results
1	Safe Zone	Meditative, relaxed, affirming, regenerative, comfortable, compassionate, peaceful	Energizing

The biggest cause of absenteeism at work is stress. Billions of pounds are lost worldwide when people are off sick. This programme identifies stress at different levels. Key factors to help identify stress in its early stages help individuals to build in strategies to counter the effects of stress before they become debilitating.

Corporate programmes

Induction class: stress rating for individuals (see Table 10.1), introduction to safety, techniques, rpm guidelines and heart rate profiles.

Heart rate profile and Emotional Zones class integration

Apprentice class (beginners)

Heart Zones 1, 2, 3 (see Fig. 4.3)
Incorporate Emotional Zones 1, 2 (see Table 7.1)
Use classes: Recovery ride and low end endurance rides 1–4 (see Fig. 6.1 to Fig. 6.5)

Business class (intermediate)

Heart Zones 1, 2, 3 (see Fig. 4.3)
Incorporate Emotional Zones 1, 2, 3 (see Table 7.1)
Use classes: Low end endurance rides 3, 4
High end endurance rides 1–4
Hill rides 1–4
Add team building (count together, ride in synchronisation)

Executive class (advanced)

Heart Zones 1, 2, 3, 4 (see Fig. 4.3)
Incorporate: Emotional Zones 1, 2, 3 (4 reactive) (see Table 7.1)
Use Classes: Low end endurance rides 3, 4
High end endurance rides 1–4
Hill rides 1–4
Extensive intervals 1
Competition 1
Team building

These are only a few examples of how you can market the classes for corporate industries; there are no boundaries – if you think of an idea, try it. The corporate world is becoming essential in terms of fitness clubs; they bring in money and people. The perfect solution for company employees is to have their own on-site gym, enabling people to join easily and train amongst friends and colleagues (as we mentioned above, joining a health club can be a trauma to some individuals). Corporate studio cycling enjoys many benefits while allowing stressed-out employees to train and get fit. At the same time we have seen that it can enhance morale and team building.

Studio cycling for teams

Having worked with some of the best clubs in the world I have been able to see that there is enormous potential for teams from many sports to benefit from studio cycling. This form of dynamic and innovative training is ideally suited to groups of people who want to train and be coached together, but still perform as individuals.

When a team member reaches a plateau, they must go back to basics to improve, which means working on simple things such as:
- Technique, mental and physical skills.
- Fitness-health, physical (cardiovascular improvement, strength, speed, power and endurance) and mental (mental health and fitness: focus, concentration to produce a 'winning mind').

Quite often an individual may need to be training at a lower level than the rest of the team and in many cases because of team spirit and peer pressure that player will overtrain as they don't want to show any weakness.

Here are some areas where we can see the benefits of studio cycling under such circumstances:

- Rehabilitation as an individual but in a team environment. The first type of exercise an injured player will do on the road to recovery will be cardiovascular training on a bike due to the load-bearing characteristics. Increasing an injured player's all-round balanced fitness can not only give a player strength and endurance but also the confidence to achieve previous form and in some cases come back stronger.

- Measuring and monitoring progress and current fitness levels. Using bikes that don't move and heart rate monitoring it will be possible to analyse a player's response to exercise.

- Advanced sports psychology. The difference between winning and losing is so small now that competitors, whether in a team or not, need to look at every possible way of gaining an edge. The difference between a winner and loser will be mental strength. In an impact sport such as football some types of training can't be done without the kind of environment that builds mental muscle. In most cases it will never have been done. We know that sports psychology works – it has been proved. How often does a football player in an important game sprint for a ball then fire wide, over the top or even scuff a shot that dribbles to the goalkeeper. Even in the World Cup a player might shoot for the goal and hit the corner flag. Nine times out of ten that player would have scored a goal in training, but with the external pressure of 70,000 screaming fans he tensed up. We can teach a player to relax under extreme pressure by focusing again and again on such critical moments with visualisation, and with the addition of a high heart rate that matches that in the game. The player will see himself score over and over until it becomes ingrained in the self-belief. Normal sports psychology works at rest, but because in studio cycling players are in one place while being physically exerted, images and ideas, thoughts and emotions can be influenced and trained.

- Team building. It can be important that this type of training takes place under extreme physical exertion with high heart rates, to build concentration, performance and synergy within the team. New players can be integrated into a team and position.

- Warm-up at side of pitch. A reserve who comes off the bench in the middle of a game needs to be ready to get into full stride immediately. The warm-up you get on a studio-cycling bike is second to none. This, with correct stretching to relax and mobilise contracting muscles, will enable a player to fly into the game.

- Team training and programming. The instructor or studio-cycling coach will liaise with the team coach or physiotherapist, or sports scientist to develop the training that the team or individuals require. This will not only build the full team but start to create an efficient support team.

- Advanced studio cycling for teams. Advanced programming for teams who have introduced studio cycling into a training regime will be to build in progressive and increased flexibility and mobility after a super-efficient warm-up on the bikes. Measurement of players' flexibility will be possible and progress developed.

If a team decides to use studio cycling in their programme they will need either to find top quality studio-cycling instructors or to train their own staff. Until now a club or team would send its players to the local health club to join in regular classes; this will not utilise the potential of a correctly run studio-cycling programme for any team.

Due to the nature of the studio-cycling warm-up and recovery phases players will recover very quickly, in some cases almost immediately, from these sessions. The recovery period prevents blood pooling and aids recycling of lactic acid, which is why studio cycling can be used as a supplement to existing physical training. Players will also use the bikes to improve recovery from other types of training and fatigue from the games themselves. This type of active recovery has long been used by competitors in multi-sport events with great success.

Below is an example of a programme run in a football or rugby club or any team sport. Some of the time frames will not coincide with current training phases, and this is because our beliefs are that studio cycling can fit on top of existing training, changing the lengths of off or close seasons and adding new training. New parts, such as the pre-season or the close season can be introduced. This vital period of time before the actual season will be an induction to the full season acclimatising players in preparation for the start.

Programme 1 (one full year including competitive season)

Designed around the team and coach requirements.

Note: this programme can only be implemented by a qualified studio-cycling Master Trainer with other core knowledge applicable to this type of training and vast experience of personal training, Heart Zone Training and studio-cycling group training for specific sports and rehabilitation.

Pre-Phase 1 (example is for football)
- Individual player assessments (physical strength and muscular endurance; psychological self-assessment and quality of focusing).
- Coach requirements, (player and team) meetings to discuss relevant information as well as observing the team in action with the coach.
- Player induction (safety, set-up, and basic techniques and positions).
- Introduction to heart rate monitoring and setting Heart Zones.

Phase 1 (close season) 1 session per week on top of normal training, 2/3 weeks in duration
- Team studio-cycling sessions (endurance).
- Squads and teams.
- Rehabilitation for any injured players.
- Backs/midfields/forwards – integration (specific to strengths and weaknesses as outlined by coaching staff).
- Introduction to mental focus exercises in Zone 2 (60–70%) of maximum.
- Flexibility upper and lower body.
- Stomach One: 6 exercises, 1–3 sets, 15–30 repetitions.
- Self-analysis and goal-setting.

Phase 2 (close season) 2–3 sessions per week on top of normal training, 4 weeks in duration
- Super-squad sessions – continue endurance training and building strength on bikes.
- Progressive flexibility extra, lower body and upper body.
- Reassessments.
- Reset goals if applicable.
- Muscular endurance exercises (weights), high repetitions.
- Stomach Two: 8 exercises, 2–4 sets, 20–30 repetitions.
- Lower back exercises × 11.

Phase 3 (pre-season) 1–2 sessions per week on top of normal training, 2 weeks in duration
- Super-team (including reserves) sessions – endurance and strength training continued, add speed and power if individuals are still improving without injury or illness (floor Heart Zone 2 to mid-point Heart Zone 4).

- Flexibility, stomach and lower back continued.
- Reassessments.

Phase 4 (season) 1 session per week on top of normal training and competitions/games

- Warm-up during games.
- Maintenance and recovery from games (mid-point Heart Zone 2.)
- Flexibility and self analyses.

Studio cycling has helped to produce some superb results in terms of sporting teams, whether it be football, rugby, netball – the list is endless. Often at some point teams or individuals find that they reach a plateau; it is then that they should go back to basics and work at a lower level than the rest of the team; in normal training this can be hard. However, with studio cycling it is impossible to know visually how hard an individual is actually working; this allows a person who has plateaued still to develop his or her training with the team and at the same time to avoid working too hard. Team training can help to rehabilitate; the instructor can work with the coach to measure and monitor an individual while allowing them to continue to train in a team environment. We have mentioned the importance of sports psychology, which helps the individuals to believe in themselves; this can also be incorporated into team-building classes where a little more competitiveness is necessary to weld the team. Studio-cycling team-building programmes will help to measure teams at various phases in their training if the coach and the studio-cycling instructor work together for mutual goals.

Training away from the bike

A *Complete Book of Studio Cycling* wouldn't *be* complete without guidelines and programmes for when you are away from the classes. 'Life out of the saddle' can be productive for a balanced training programme. It is not a good idea to do only studio cycling as this can lead to monotony, which will reflect in your training and in your teaching if you are planning classes. In life we must have balance and multi-sport training is certainly more balanced and healthy.

This book is not attempting to dictate how many classes you should do a week; however, if you want to make a difference to your fitness, improve your outdoor cycling or lose weight, we advocate that you should try studio cycling 2–3 times a week. If possible the classes should generally be higher intensity; however, the beauty of studio cycling is that you are able to ride according to how you feel.

Studio cycling enables participants to warm up and recover the body efficiently because we can raise the core temperature of the body and muscles before we elevate the heart rate. While recovering, the core temperature stays high while the heart rate decreases, reducing blood pooling and recycling lactic acid. This procedure means that there isn't the localised soreness as with other, impact exercises such as running, aerobics etc. If you have your own schedule then ideally you should place studio cycling as one of the hard efforts of the week; however, if cycling is not your sole goal or sport it can also be used as a great recovery exercise.

Everyone is different and responds individually to exercise, so what works for one will not work for another. Therefore there will need to be a certain element of coaching input for interpreting the responses.

It would be useful to include an element of resistance exercises. You can follow this programme for an excellent balanced schedule in addition to your studio-cycling work-outs. Does it fit in with goals you have set yourself in the ten steps?

Fig. 7.2   Resistance – upper body

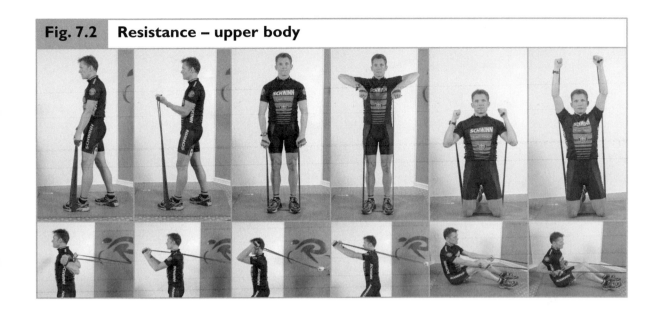

Fig. 7.3   Resistance – lower body

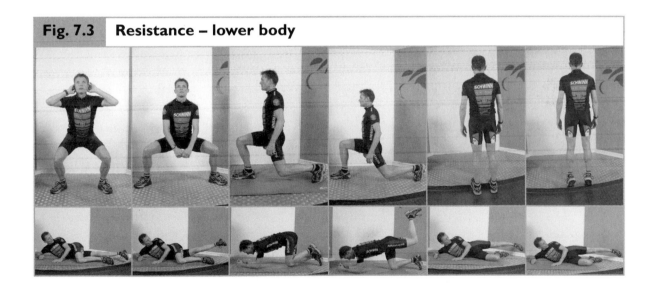

Table 7.2	Example of 4-week training diary		
Week I	**Morning**	**Midday**	**Afternoon**
Monday			Studio cycling – low end endurance class (LEE) Zone 2–3
Tuesday		Walk – 30 minutes Zone 1<2	Weights – upper body 2/3 sets and 10<20 reps (5 exercises)
Wednesday			Studio cycling – hill class Zone 3<4
Thursday	Rest day		
Friday			Studio cycling – LEE
Saturday	Long slow walk/jog/run (1 hour+) Zone 2		
Sunday	Rest day		
Week 2	**Morning**	**Midday**	**Afternoon**
Monday			Studio cycling – low end endurance class (LEE) Zone 2<3
Tuesday		Walk – 35 minutes Zone 1<2	Weights – upper body 2/3 sets and 15<20 reps (5 exercises)
Wednesday			Studio cycling – hill class Zone 3<4
Thursday	Rest day		
Friday			Studio cycling – high end endurance class Zones 3–4
Saturday	Long slow jog/run (1 hour 15 minutes) Zone 2		
Sunday	Rest day		
Week Three	**Morning**	**Midday**	**Afternoon**
Monday	2 x 20 press-ups 2 x 30 sit-ups		Studio cycling – low end endurance class (LEE). Zone 2<3
Tuesday		Walk – 40 minutes Zone 1<2	Weights – upper body 3/4 sets and 20 reps (5 exercises)

Wednesday			Studio cycling – hill class Zone 3<4
Thursday	Rest day		
Friday			Studio cycling – competition class Zone 3<5 Weights – lower body (5 exercises)
Saturday	Long slow walk/jog/run (1 hour 30 minutes) Zone 2		
Sunday	Rest day		
Week Four	**Morning**	**Midday**	**Afternoon**
Monday	40 press-ups 3 × 30 sit-ups		Studio cycling – low end endurance class (LEE) Zone 2<3
Tuesday		Walk – 40 minutes Zone 1<2	Weights – upper body 4 sets and 20 reps (6 exercises)
Wednesday			Studio cycling – competition class Zone 3<4
Thursday	Run 30 minutes Zone 2/3 (include 15 minutes at tempo pace – Zone 4)		
Friday			Studio cycling – LEE Zone 2<3 Weights – upper and lower body (as before)
Saturday	Long slow jog/run (2 hours) Zone 2		
Sunday	Rest day		

Instructor tip:

Some sports-specific athletes can use studio cycling as threshold work – Zone 4<5

Advanced stretching: PNF stretches

In the studio-cycling class programme we have concentrated on basic stretches that can be done beside the bike. In this section we introduce longer, slower, deeper stretches that you will have more time and space for. Show these to your classes so they can do them on their own. Include PNF stretches.

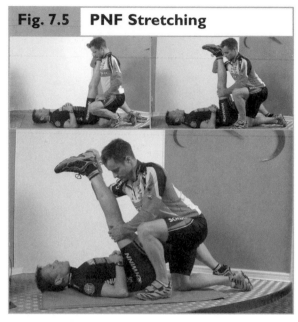

Fig. 7.5 PNF Stretching

Calf stretches

Stretch the calf by pushing the ball of the foot into the ground for 5 seconds then releasing it, then continue the stretch. If the leg is tight you are overstretching – don't go any further. If it can go further with no tightness continue. Do each stretch three times with each leg.

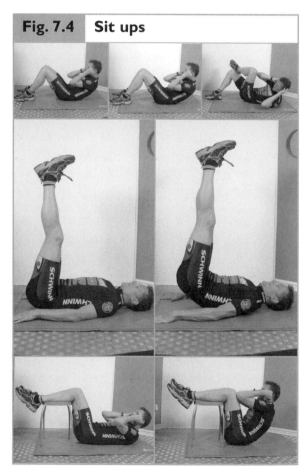

Fig. 7.4 Sit ups

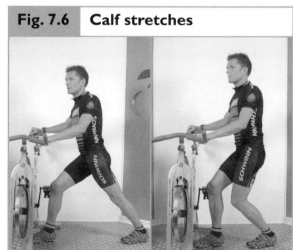

Fig. 7.6 Calf stretches

STUDIO CYCLING AT HOME

8

This chapter is for the benefit of those people who have a studio-cycling bike at home. Your bike doesn't have to have a fixed flywheel; as long as you can set the bike up correctly and safely then you can follow the programme set out for you here. Use the same principles of training progression and motivating techniques as in the rest of the book.

The following programme is designed to motivate you through sound progressive exercise principles, measuring progress and adding intensities and durations, as they are needed. Spend just a few minutes familiarising yourself with the programme. You will find the meaning of any unfamiliar terms in the Glossary at the end of the book. Once you understand it will be as easy as pedalling!

Pick a selection of your favourite music, to last between 30 minutes and 1 hour. Mix slow and fast music to match with the programmes.

Visualisation

Visualisation can be used to picture somewhere you want to ride or to imagine a positive experience connected with your life – it can be anything good! You can use the music to help

you have a strong visualisation. A slow beat of music can evoke a climb; fast beats can signify flat roads or descents. Be imaginative!

PHASE ONE – beginners to intermediate

This phase should be completed within 4 weeks approximately (see Table 8.1).

Intensity levels

There are three ways to measure the level of intensity: revolutions per minute (rpm), rate of perceived exertion (RPE) or, as we recommend, the use of HRM (heart rate monitoring). If you do not have a heart rate monitor and don't wish to buy one then please use RPE. In Phase Two you will need a heart rate monitor.

1 **Revolutions per minute (rpm)** – rpm = cadence, or how many times the pedals go round in 1 minute. During the programme you can monitor your rpm and relate the efforts in comparison to the heart rate.
2 **RPE, scale 1–10** – represents the level you think you are at. Try to match how you feel to the levels given in the programme: 1 = very easy pace; 5–7 = warm-up; 7–8.5 = aerobic 8.5–9.5 = hard; 10 = very hard.
3 **Training heart rates** – find maximum heart rate – see Chapter 4 on Heart Zone Training.

Visualisation examples:

- The best race of your life
- Scoring a goal (perfect technique)
- Hitting the bull's-eye
- Making love
- Winning
- Your favourite ride

Find % of maximum and record in this space	
Average resting heart rate =	RPE = 1
50% =	RPE = 5
60% =	RPE = 6
70% =	RPE = 7
75% =	RPE = 7.5
80% =	RPE = 8
85% =	RPE = 8.5
90% =	RPE = 9
95% =	RPE = 9.5
Max. =	RPE = 10

Before you begin

- Check your bike – see bike maintenance manual from manufacturer if you are not sure.
- Understand – the fixed-gear principle of spinning without freewheeling if you are using this type of bike.
- Make sure you are comfortable with the fit.
- Sizing – saddle (up/down/forward/aft) – see diagrams on bike set-up in Chapter 2.
- Handlebars (up/down).
- Pick a selection of your favourite music to last between 30 minutes and 1 hour.

Work-out rules

- Make sure you have water and a towel!
- Key your first track and start pedalling. Use low resistance/gear 70–90 rpms.

1 Note – always allow plenty of time to recover from the previous ride. If you are training for an event, make sure your visualisation is positive and matches your goal.
2 Stretch after each warm-up or at the end of every warm-down. This will help to prevent injury.

To complete Phase Two you will need the following:

- Heart rate monitor
- Carbohydrate drink
- Music that motivates you.

Phase Two – Intermediate

Information on Phase Two at home

Now you are entering into Phase Two you must take into account some further important considerations to aid your improvement (see Table 8.2).

1 Diet – what you eat and when.
2 Nutrition – supplementation for the individual (See Chapter 1, under Nutrition).
3 Rest and recovery – fit a training schedule around your lifestyle and allow plenty of time off to relax.
4 Focus, balance and consistency – if you have difficulty in doing this you may want to consider being coached.
5 Refer to ride A, B, C, and D but start to add distance, speed and time.

Important:
- Do not move on to Phase Two until you have successfully completed all of Phase One.
- Use the same heart rate % in Phase Two that you worked out for Phase One.

Phase Three (10 turbo sessions)

Only when you have completed Phase Two will you be ready to move on to Phase Three where we can assume you can focus and concentrate for long periods of time. You are motivated and have seen the results from the previous two phases and are willing to do the next ten sessions in three weeks+ fitting them into the rest of your training and goals. Most of the sessions are self-explanatory, but the turbo session 4 requires a little more instruction.

Table. 8.1	Phase One

Phase One – Week 1 ride A

(complete this ride twice in 1st week, then move on to ride B at start of 2nd week)

Ride to the rhythm of your music or count rpms.

Warm-up. 5 minutes spinning at 80–90 rpm, heart rate – 60<70% or RPE 6<7

Visualisation. 5 minutes at 90 rpm, heart rate – 70<75% or RPE 7>7.5

Visualisation. 10 minutes at 90 rpm, heart rate – 75>85% or RPE 7.5>8.5

Change gear/add resistance. 10 minutes at 90 rpm, heart rate – 85% or RPE 8.5

Warm-down. 5 minutes at 90–80 RPM

Stretch. 5 minutes

Total time = 40 minutes

Phase One – Week 2 add ride B

(complete this ride 2–3 times but put ride A in between)

Warm-up. 5 minutes spinning at 80–90 rpm, heart rate – 60-70% or RPE 6<7

Main set:

Seated climb (visualisation). 3 minutes at 70 rpm, heart rate – 70<85% or RPE 7<8.5

Combination flat/jumps. 1 minute – with the rhythm, same rates as above

Standing climb (visualisation). 3 minutes, same rates as above

Spin recovery. 3 minutes at 90 rpm, heart rate – 65%

Important: Don't go above 85% during main set – *repeat main set three times*

Warm-down. 5 minutes spinning at 90>60 rpm, heart rate – 85>60%

Stretch. 5 minutes

Total time = 45 minutes (add more main sets if this is too easy)

Phase One – Week 3 add ride C

(complete this ride 3 times but alternate it with ride B in third week)

Long visualisation. Warm-up stay seated. 15 minutes spinning at 70<100 rpm, heart rate – 60<75%

Seated climb (visualisation). 10 minutes at 70 rpm, heart rate – 75<85% gradually, with resistance

Descend. 2 minutes at 100 rpm, heart rate – 85>65% or where it falls to after 2 minutes

Seated flat. 10 minutes at 100 rpm, heart rate – 75<80%

Descend. 2 minutes at 110 rpm, heart rate – 80>70%

Standing climb. 5 minutes at 60 rpm, heart rate – 85%

Warm-down. 5 minutes spinning at 90>50 rpm

Stretch. 5 minutes

Total time = 54 minutes (endurance day)

Phase One – Week 4 add ride D

(complete this ride twice alternating with ride C then B then move on to next phase)

Warm-up. 5 minutes at 100 rpm, heart rate – 60<70%

Main set:

Standing. 5 × 1 minute with 30 seconds in saddle between at 85 rpm, heart rate – 75<80%
Sitting. 5 minutes at 95 rpm, heart rate – 85%
Combination flat/jump. 5 × 10 (10 every 45 seconds approx.) at 75<95 rpm, heart rate – 85%

Repeat main set twice

Warm-down. 5 minutes at 120>80 rpm, heart rate – 85>65%
Stretch. 5 minutes

Total time = 45 minutes

Table. 8.2 Phase Two

Phase Two – Week 1 ride A

(complete this ride twice in 1st week – then move on to ride B at start of 2nd week)

Ride to the rhythm of your music or count rpms

Warm-up. 10 minutes spinning at 80–90 rpm, heart rate – 60<70% or RPE 6<7

Visualisation. 5 minutes at 90 rpm, heart rate – 70<75% or RPE 7<7.5

Visualisation. 10 minutes at 90 rpm, heart rate – 75<85% or RPE 7.5<8.5

Change gear/add resistance. 10 minutes at 90 rpm, heart rate – 85% or RPE 8.5

Warm-down. 10 minutes at 90>80 RPM

Stretch. 5 minutes

Total time = 50 minutes

Phase Two – Week 2 add ride B

(complete this ride 2–3 times but put ride A in between)

Warm-up. 10 minutes spinning at 80–90 rpm, heart rate – 60-70% or RPE 6<7

Main set:

Seated climb (visualisation). 3 minutes at 70 rpm, heart rate – 75<85% or RPE 7<8.5

Combination hills/jumps. 1 minute – slow rhythm as you feel and with the rhythm, heart rate 85<90%

Standing climb (visualisation) 3 minutes – same rates as above

Spin recovery for 2 minutes at 90 rpm, heart rate – 70%

Important: don't go above 90% during main set – *repeat main set 5 times*

Warm-down. 5 minutes spinning at 90>60 rpm, heart rate – 90>60%

Stretch. 5 minutes

Total time = 65 minutes

Phase Two – Week 3 add ride C

(complete this ride 3 times but alternate it with ride B in third week with one A ride optional)

Long visualisation – warm-up. Stay seated 15 minutes spinning at 80<120 rpm, heart rate – 60<80%

Seated climb (visualisation). 10 minutes at 70 rpm, heart rate – 80<85% gradually with resistance.

Descend. 1 minute at 120 rpm, heart rate – 85>70% or where it falls to after 1 min. (RECORD DROP)

Seated flat. 15 minutes at 100 rpm, heart rate – 80<85%

Descend. 1 minute at 125 rpm, heart rate – 85>70% or where heart rate falls to after 1 min. (RECORD DROP)

Standing climb. 15 minutes at 60<70 rpm, heart rate – 85%

Warm-down. 10 minutes spinning at 90>50 rpm

Stretch. 5 minutes

Total time = 72 minutes (endurance day)

Phase Two – Week 4 add ride D

(complete this ride twice alternating with ride C then B and A then move on to next phase)

Warm-up. 10 minutes at 100 rpm, heart rate – 60<75%

Main set:

Standing. 5 × 1 minute with 30 seconds in saddle in between at 85 rpm, heart rate – 80<85%

Sitting. 5 minutes at 95 rpm, heart rate – 90%

Combination flat/jump. 5 × 20 jumps (20 every 45 seconds approx.) at 75<95 rpm, heart rate – 85<95%

Repeat main set 3 times

Warm-down. 10 minutes at 120>80 rpm, heart rate – 85>65%

Stretch. 5 minutes

Total time = 73 minutes

Table. 8.3	Turbo work-out 1 (45 minutes approximately)

Warm-up. Spin the legs for 5 minutes in a high gear/easy resistance, 95<100 rpm

Set 1:
    5 × 20 seconds each leg in same gear/resistance as warm-up
    Drop down a gear/add resistance and repeat
    Drop down a gear/add resistance and repeat
    Spin legs at 120 rpm for 2–3 minutes

Set 2:
    4 × 1 minute – low gear/heavy resistance (30 seconds recovery between)
    2 minutes spin recovery between
    4 × 1 minute – lower gear/heavier resistance (45 seconds recovery between)
    2 minutes spin recovery
    4 × 1 minute – lower gear/heavier resistance (1 minute recovery between)

Warm-down. Spin legs for 5 minutes (90<110 rpm)
Full stretch. 5<10 minutes

Record this information to add to your logbook later:	
Dates completed:	
Starting heart rate at rest:	
Time spent:	
How I felt:	
Recovery heart rate at end of work-out:	

Table. 8.4	Turbo work-out 2 (40–45 minutes approximately)

Warm-up. Spin legs in high gear/light resistance for 10 minutes

Set 1.
   6 × 2 minutes with progressive heart rate e.g. 70–85 % of maximum heart rate or aerobic to anaerobic threshold
   1 minute spin legs recovery

Set 2.
20 × 20 seconds each leg – alternate (do this in aerodynamic position)

Warm-down. Spin legs 100+ for 10 minutes
Full stretch. 5<10 minutes

Record this information to add to your logbook later:

Dates completed:

Starting heart rate at rest:

Time spent:

How I felt:

Recovery heart rate at end of work-out:

Table. 8.5	Turbo work-out 3 (45–50 minutes approximately)

Warm-up. Spin legs for 5<10 minutes in high gear/light resistance at 90<100 rpm

Set 1.
   5 × 5 minutes building from aerobic to anaerobic pace (use your Heart Rate Chart)
   30 seconds recovery, slow spin in between

Set 2.
   5 × 100 rpl (revolutions per leg) medium gearing/resistance (alternating legs)

Warm up. Spin legs for 5<10 minutes easy
Full stretch. 5<10 minutes

Record this information to add to your logbook later:

Dates completed:

Starting heart rate at rest:

Time spent:

How I felt:

Recovery heart rate at end of work-out:

Turbo work-out 4 (TEN-MILE TIME TRIAL)

(40–50 minutes approximately)

You will need a bike computer, heart rate monitor and Turbo Trainer. Set the turbo trainer so that the back wheel is only just touching the flywheel when you are sitting on the bike. You can calibrate this so that it is always the same by pedalling up to 15 mph then stopping and counting the revolutions of the wheel or noting the time it takes to stop. This becomes your benchmark gear and resistance each time you do this trial.

Warm-up. 5<10 minutes at 95<110 rpm (RPE = 5–7 or heart rate = 50<70% of max HR)

Set clock and trip distance to zero, make sure you have a heart rate reading.

Find a suitable gearing to allow you to spin the pedals at 120 rpm, then start the clock and trip distance.

You must record the:
- Time
- Heart rate
- Gear used – EACH MILE FOR 10 MILES
- rpm if unable to reach 120.

Have a pen and paper in place to record this information while you go. You may need someone to do this for you.

This is a continuous 10-MILE time trial at 120 rpm (if possible).

Table. 8.6	Turbo work-out 4 (cont.) (10 Mile Time Trial (holding 120 rpms))		
Date........................ Gear .... /Resistance .... Starting Heart Rate at Rest			
Miles	Mile times	rpm/speed	Heart rates
1			
2			
3			
4			
5			
6			
7			
8			
9			
10			

Table. 8.7	Turbo work-out 5 (50 minutes approximately)

Work out your max heart rate before you start (see Chapter 4); use a reliable heart monitor

Warm-up. 5-10 minutes – keep your heart rate at low aerobic range but high 90+ rpm

Set 1 (keep cadence at 90+ rpm)
  4 × 1 min at 75% of max HR
  10 seconds between spin recovery
  4 × 1 min at 80% of max HR
  15 seconds between spin recovery
  4 × 1 min at 85% of max HR
  20 seconds between spin recovery
  4 × 1 min at 90% of max HR
  20 seconds between spin recovery

Recovery after Set 1. 5 minutes of alternate one-leg drills of your choice

Set 2
  30 seconds at 85%
  15 seconds spin recovery
  45 seconds at 85%
  25 seconds spin recovery
  60 seconds at 85%
  1 minute easy recovery
  Repeat at 90%
  Repeat at 95%
  Repeat at 100%

Full stretch off the bike. Warm-down spin 10 minutes.

Record this information to add to your logbook later:

Dates completed:

Starting heart rate at rest:

Time spent:

How I felt:

Recovery heart rate at end of work-out:

Table. 8.8	Turbo work-out 6 (75 minutes approximately)

Warm-up. 5–10 minutes. Gradually increase your heart rate from resting to 75% of max.

Set 1
   5 min at 75% heart rate – 120 rpm
   5 min at 80% heart rate – 120 rpm
   5 min at 85% heart rate – 120 rpm
   5 min at 90% heart rate – 120 rpm
   5 min at 95% heart rate – 120 rpm
   5 min at 95% heart rate – 120 rpm
   5 minutes easy recovery

Set 2
   5 min at 80% heart rate – 120 rpm
   5 min at 85% heart rate – 120 rpm
   5 min at 90% heart rate – 120 rpm
   15 min at 80 – 85% heart rate – 85<100 rpm

Warm down.
Full stretch.

Record this information to add to your logbook later:

Dates completed:

Starting heart rate at rest:

Time spent:

How I felt:

Recovery heart rate at end of work-out:

Table. 8.9	Turbo work-out 7 (90 minutes approximately)

Warm-up. Spinning with high cadence for 10 minutes, getting heart rate above 70% of max or 130 bpm approximately.

Work in an aerodynamic position:
10 minutes at 19 mph
3 minutes at 22 mph
5 minutes at 20 mph
3 minutes at 23 mph

Repeat above work × 3 (add 1–2 mph if these speeds are too easy)
Gradually look for a gears change – used as you grow in strength
Warm-down. 5 minutes easy (including one-leg spinning)
Full stretch off the bike

Record this information to add to your logbook later:

Dates completed:

Starting heart rate at rest:

Time spent:

How I felt:

Recovery heart rate at end of work-out:

Table. 8.10	Turbo work-out 8 (45 minutes approximately)

Warm-up. 10 minutes – gently raise heart rate to 140 bpm or 75–80% of max

Work:
5 × (2 minutes at 23 mph or 85% + 1 min at 25 mph or 90%)
Recovery. 3 minutes spin

Work:
10 minutes alternating left and right leg (do a pyramid: 30L – 30R, 35L – 35R, 40L – 40R, etc. up to 100 each leg.

Warm-down. Easy for 5 minutes

Record this information to add to your logbook later:

Dates completed:

Starting heart rate at rest:

Time spent:

How I felt:

Recovery heart rate at end of work-out:

Table. 8.11	Turbo work-out 9 (1 hour approximately)

Warm-up. 10 minutes – raise heart rate to 70% of max

Work:
3 × (7 minutes at 80%, 3 minutes at 85%, 1 minute at 90–95%)
Recovery. 3 minutes spin easy
5 minutes high cadence 100<120+ rpm
Warm-down. As you like for 5 minutes, including:
Full stretch off the bike

Record this information to add to your logbook later:

Dates completed:

Starting heart rate at rest:

Time spent:

How I felt:

Recovery heart rate at end of work-out:

Table. 8.12	Turbo work-out 10 (35–40 minutes approximately)

Warm-up. Ramping up mph or kph:
   I minute for each speed registered on computer
   Start easy or 15 mph – Repeat at 16, 17, 18, 19, 20, 21, 22, 23, 24, 25, 26, 27, 28, go as high as you can
   Record your heart rates for each speed, so that when you repeat this test you can compare them.
You will need to calibrate the Turbo Trainer for accuracy. (See Turbo work-out 4.)

Record this information to add to your logbook later:

Dates completed:

Starting heart rate at rest:

Time spent:

How I felt:

Recovery heart rate at end of work-out:

ATHLETES 'SPIN TO WIN'

You can see the results of a studio-cycling programme with the individuals whose goals are general, such as weight loss, cardiovascular improvements and general fitness in short periods of time. This chapter is devoted to sportsmen and -women or athletes who train and compete in sports other than cycling but can benefit from it. You can use studio cycling as an addition to your existing schedule. A consistent regime of studio cycling can benefit your sport.

Cyclists and triathletes 'spin to win'

If you watch professional cyclists in the top races such as the Tour de France you will see that although they are incredibly fit, look very comfortable and ride at amazing speeds, a few riders are not showing perfect technique with their upper body. This is because they don't have to teach others. A studio-cycling instructor must lead by example, otherwise those who follow will copy poor technique. So cyclists don't have to have perfect technique, but as a coach this could be an area you could help them in. You may be more qualified to help cyclists than they are, or even than their coach. A cyclist will find it simple to fit in a studio-cycling programme because, obviously, cycling is his or her sport. However, most cyclists tend to neglect the one aspect to their cycling that will give them the best benefits – balance to their training. The low end and high end endurance rides are easiest for them but the 45–60 minute threshold rides are often missing.

(See Class Profiles, Chapter 6: Extensive Intervals, Intensive Intervals, Competition Classes etc.) Just two classes a week can make the difference within 4–5 weeks. If cyclists add this training into their workouts for 2 months during the winter, by the spring they will be ready to race.

This also works the other way: if a studio cyclist is going to race they must do the longer steady rides to help build the strength and endurance that is missing from the classes. In reality we don't have the time to spin for 2–3 hours in the studio.

Other sports

Studio cycling will work for most sports, as 1–2 rides can be added to almost any heavy schedule because it is load-bearing and the recovery is so complete. The classes can be used for active recovery from any sports training. Most rides will only need to be recovery, with low and high end endurance used if appropriate, leaving specificity of training to the actual sport. However, if you have an injury that prohibits you doing your chosen sport then of course you can choose the class profiles that will work the correct fitness elements of endurance, strength, speed and power.

OVERTRAINING

10

Symptoms of overtraining must be identified in the early stages in order to prevent illness and injury. They appear in the form of chronic fatigue and infection, as it is possible that the immune system becomes depressed.

There will always be positive and negative effects to training. You can use the information below to help you coach yourself and others. Decide if any of the symptoms are present and look at how to build in the recovery needed. Studio cyclists will often overtrain due to the euphoric feelings they get after a class.

In terms of heart rate response, overtraining will show up in raised ambient, delta and resting heart rate. There is no set increased number, although you must have a previous record of your 'normal' resting heart rate, so that you can gauge and record the increase. If your resting heart rate is 10 beats or higher than your normal resting heart rate you must train in the lower zones. See Heart Zones, Chapter 4, for more details.

There are other signs to look out for, give yourself an OS (Overtraining and Stress) rating; look at the scale below and give a number to each symptom. The number can also correspond to the increase in ambient, resting and delta heart rate, which you can include in the rating. Try to rate at least ten symptoms, which means you will include one heart rate factor. Other than the heart rate indicators there are some positives to having a degree of extra stress, but once you rate more than 5 look out for overtraining.

You can repeat this test monthly with your clients and yourself. An interesting pattern may emerge which will enable you to adjust training accordingly. Although you may not want to give it to all your class members it may be valuable for someone who needs a little extra coaching as he or she isn't responding positively to your class.

Balance

To balance your training with adequate recovery becomes as much an artform as a science. This is another good reason to advocate multi-sport training. A really motivated individual is likely to train hard all the time or too frequently. An intense studio-cycling class on day 1, followed by a weight training session, could fatigue the body enough to ensure slower recovery. If you were to attempt to repeat the previous day's exercise the OS rating may go up by several points. This is a form of over-reaching, which can be positive as long as you include recovery. Instead of no training at all an easy session in low Heart Zones 1 or 2 could be all that is needed. For people who want or need to train every day, another type of sport could be used, such as swimming (load-bearing), rowing (load-bearing) or running at low end endurance (impact).

FITT (frequency, intensity, time and type)

This is where coaching really comes into its own and how you use the FITT formula within your lifestyle will have a bearing on your success. (See Heart Zones, Chapter 4.)

Table. 10.1	Overtraining and stress analysis (OS)	

Overtraining/stress analysis rating 1–10
    1 = Relaxed
    2 = Normal
    3 = Involved
    4 = Concentrated
    5 = Very involved
    6 = Tense
    7 = Unsettled
    8 = Fatigued
    9 = Struggling
   10 = Very overtrained

Previous scores	Symptoms	Today's rating 1–10
	• Tiredness	
	• Lethargy	
	• Insomnia	
	• Irritability	
	• Depression	
	• Flatulence	
	• Diarrhoea	
	• Clamminess	
	• Night sweats	
	• Anxiety	
	• Frequent urination	
	• Loss of appetite	
	• Loss of interest in sex	
	• Resting heart rate	
	• Ambient heart rate	
	• Delta heart rate	
Total		

Rest and recovery

The harder you train, the more your body will need to sleep. Sleeping is the best form of rest but sometimes just having a day off from training, or training in a lower Heart Zone will be adequate. During sleep the body can restore itself, repair and recover. Without this vital recovery the next training session will be a negative experience, it will hurt more than normal, leaving you frustrated and tired. This negative feeling will be the thing you remember when you come to plan your next session, and could persuade you not to do it!

Other forms of recovery come in the form of:
• **Active recovery** – Zone 1 light level cardiovascular activity such as spinning the legs with very little resistance for an extended period, followed by deep stretches when the muscles are warm.

- **Stretching** – can be done before, during and after work-outs; however, the length and depth of the stretches will vary depending on goals and time. Be progressive with longer, slower, deeper stretches. Use the breathing rule (see flexibility).
- **Massage** – self-massage is therapeutic, it will pick up potential stiffness and help you find key areas that may be tightening up, thus needing extra work before they turn into an injury. Nevertheless, a perfect solution to sore and tight muscles is a good sports massage. When someone else massages you, they can pick up a lot more than if you do it yourself.
- **Saunas** – the Scandinavians organise a whole social scene around saunas; however, they are not just good for socialising they are also great for tired muscles, and can really relax them and aid recovery. Be sure to hydrate enough though, especially after an exhausting and hot class, take a drink in with you.
- **Jacuzzis** – are a great way to unwind. Heat and water jets that can be angled into the muscles.

Be open-minded to natural therapies, they can be incredibly effective and speed recovery from exercise and injury.

You should not train in a normal studio-cycling class if the following factors apply:
- High OS rating (see Table 10.1)
- High blood pressure
- Injury
- Illness
- On certain medications.

Illness and injury

If you train too hard without recovering your immune system, all the hard work will be wasted. By getting ill or injured you will be forced into inactivity and lose the fitness that you have built up and worked for.

Overtraining is not always easy to spot, or rather most people would sooner not admit to it! By now you will be able to see more clearly whether or not you are working your body too hard; if you are suffering sleepless nights, fatigue and loss of appetite you could be one of the people we have discussed. Perhaps the most important thing is recognising that you are overtrained, and discovering the best way to allow your body to recover and adapt to the exercise that you need. The OS rating and the heart rate guidelines above will give you an indication of whether or not your body is ready. If you are pregnant and have been active before, then you will need to keep a careful watch on your volume of exercise as well as your heart rate; the same applies to people undergoing a cardiac (cardio rehab) rehabilitation programme. Do not ignore the signs of overtraining, they are your body's way of trying to tell you something; work with your body and it will work with you, allowing you to reach those important goals.

SPECIAL POPULATIONS

11

Pregnancy

There will be times when a pregnant woman wants to train. There are a lot of reasons why she should, and much that could hinder her training. Generally a pregnant woman will be in touch with her GP and be taking advice. Quite a lot of information is available now and in most cases light exercise is recommended and even prescribed. Regular monitoring is advised, however, as in pregnancy things can change as a woman moves through her trimesters. High blood pressure is a cause for concern and only the lightest of exercise is recommended. An advanced studio-cycling class should be avoided because it is too easy to get carried away. An instructor could consider giving the client a heart monitor so she can use guidelines such as that 65–70% of max is the hardest she should work. Be aware though that every pregnant woman will be different. It would be only sensible to ask a pregnant woman to sign a waiver form before the class.

Pregnancy guidelines
- Limit of leg speed, 60–100 rpm.
- Heart rate for first period of pregnancy, 65–75% of max (for predicted max see tests in Chapter 4, Heart Zones).
- Heart rate for second phase, 65–70% of max.
- Clients with high blood pressure 55–65% of max.

Rehabilitation from injury

In some cases the only exercise a person who has an injury will be able to do is cycling, because it is load-bearing. If the injury doesn't hurt when cycling then this will be an excellent exercise to maintain and even build cardiovascular and muscular endurance. However, an instructor must help the participant decide whether to attend the class or use the studio-cycling bike on their own or in a one-to-one situation. If, as the instructor, you are unsure of the individual's motivation, you may be able to work one to one with them or place them on a programme with someone who is also injured or recovering from illness; even an unconditioned person may be the ideal training partner.

Their programme will need supervision and regular monitoring to ensure the rate of progress is constant. Just as with the regular class schedule, there must be challenges and progression built in. Some people become very despondent and unmotivated when they cannot train in their usual sport or at their usual intensity. Talk to them; tell them that this is a positive therapy and will speed up their rehabilitation by 100%. In many cases injured people have come back to their chosen sport stronger and more motivated after following a consistent programme such as with the studio-cycling bikes.

Cardio rehabilitation

Anyone who has had a heart attack, or other heart-related problems or a stroke will be very worried when they elevate their heart rate for the first time after their illness. This is to be expected. There are many considerations a studio-cycling coach or personal trainer will need to know, and one is that studio cycling is probably the best form of exercise a cardio rehab patient could take, because it is load-bearing, the bikes don't move, and the heavy, uncalibrated flywheel can be pedalled with very little resistance and is micro-adjustable. As long as the motor skills have not been impaired, it is an ideal form of exercise. However, the class format will not be applicable unless there is a group of similar patients, because exercise with unimpaired individuals would be a daunting prospect and not supportive of rehabilitation.

Classes are being specially designed for people who are at risk of heart-related diseases known as 'Heart zones pre-event classes' (an 'event' is a stroke or heart attack). The classes take into account risk factors such as a sedentary lifestyle, obesity, high blood pressure, elevated stress levels, age and history of hereditary disease.

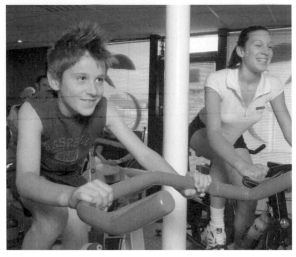

children and younger people.

These days more children than ever lead a sedentary lifestyle. This negative trend can lead to obesity and cardiovascular disease in the upcoming adult population. It is vital we target this group for education through fun, energetic pursuits such as studio cycling so that the positive results they see and feel inspire and motivate them to want to lead an active and healthy life.

Just like adults, juniors respond to change and gain satisfaction and motivation from positive changes – but we must never assume they are just small adults. Some important differences will be in the field of fitness and health, but we

Juniors

In this section we will look at studio cycling programming and recommendations for

Table. 11.1	Guidelines and recommendations for rating level of exercise by problem			
Type of heart problem	rpm	Heart rates	RPE	Cycling techniques
Heart attack	50–70	50–60%	5<6	Seated flat
Stroke	50–70	50–65%	5<6.5	Seated flat and climb
Double bypass	50–75	50–65%	5<6.5	Seated flat
Triple bypass	50–70	50–65%	5<6.5	Seated flat
Quadruple bypass	50–65	50–65%	5<6.5	Seated flat
Pacemaker	60–110	50–80%	5<8	Seated flat, climb, standing climb
Medications	60–90	50–70%	5<7	Seated flat, climb

need also to foster higher levels of concentration, especially in long-term students. Children and adolescents need exercise for physical growth but also for psychological development. Studies have shown that for children long periods of inactivity can result in diminished motor activity.

However, we need to look for simple and key factors that will be more effective and show tangible results for this unique and special population group, and we must focus on personal improvements rather than measuring a child's performance against that of his or her peers, as this can be devastating for a junior who works hard but is never as good as someone else. Tools like the studio-cycling bike that has no calibrated resistance to measure one performance against another, and the heart rate monitor that measures individual performance, can teach young people that they are all winners.

Studio-cycling classes for juniors have to be fun as their attention span is short to start with. Initially they will perceive boredom as a problem, and just getting them onto the bikes will be difficult. There are many ways that this exercise can be delivered that will still give the fun and exciting elements but also administer a progressive programme from a coaching perspective.

The premise of 'what works for one child will work for another' is often mistakenly thought to be acceptable. This is not the case, and so each child will need to be introduced gently to guidelines, which will include legs speeds (cadence), pace change with resistance and a basic introduction to heart rate monitoring as a positive, fun and educational programme.

One goal of this programme should be to engender positive behaviour from increasing self-worth, encouraging young people to see how unlimited their potential is! The overall health and well-being of a child or junior can be determined not just from their appearance and performance, but more importantly from their self-image and self-worth.

To put principles into practice, follow the junior studio-cycling programme, which sets simple guidelines and easy techniques to take children to a new physical and psychological level of development.

Growth in children

Growth in children is not linear but irregular and the first phase of puberty, where some children may be tall enough to ride the studio-cycling bikes, would normally start at around 10 years old for early developers. Normally girls are a little ahead of boys as you can see in the developmental stages in relationship to chronological age.

In the British Schools Cycling Association (BSCA) children are encouraged to ride as young as under 8 years old, with age categories of under-10s and under-12s. However, strict guidelines must be observed and these three age groups must ride bikes with free wheels (not fixed wheels as with studio-cycling bikes). Record attempts for the under-14s must not exceed one hour. Record attempts for the under-12s must not exceed 30 minutes, and record attempts for under-10s will not be recognised. Also there are strict guidelines for gear restrictions. The maximum gear will be the distance covered per crank revolution of 5.1 metres for under-8s, 5.4 metres for under-10s, 6.3 metres for under-12s, 6.4 metres for the under-14s, 6.9 metres for the under-16s and 17.3 metres for the over-16s. Heavy regulation on distances of races are also set. Under-8s will race no more than 3 km; under-10s, 5 km; under-12s, 10 km; under-14s, 20 km; under-16s, 35 km; and above 16 years old will be at the organisers' discretion. Of course these are for distance events and there are many more events, such as pursuits etc. that have other recommendations. Mountain-bike competitions use time restrictions of 15 minutes plus one lap for under-8s up to 40 minutes plus one lap for under-16s. These restrictions ensure that children are not overextending themselves, risking health problems as they get older. We should examine BSCA guidelines for children and apply them to our studio-cycling classes so that we can use similar times and distances for our children's programmes, while ensuring safe and effective classes.

During pre-puberty the focus is primarily on coordination and memory.

1st Phase of puberty	girls 11/12–13/14
(youths)	boys 12/13–14/15

In this phase children begin to detach themselves from parental influence and start to question authority. They want to do things of their own and need to be allowed to. They want to spend more time with their peers. An instructor coach will recognise this and introduce classes as team-building exercises not led by the instructor but by rules, games and guidelines agreed on together. This will enhance harmony through mutual respect and the games will involve democratic expression with everyone allowed a chance to lead the group. Aim to improve physical attributes first and coordination secondary.

2nd Phase of puberty	girls 13/14–17/18
(juniors)	boys 14/15–18/19

This stage marks the start of adolescence, the final phase of growth before adulthood. Growth starts to slow down. They are now ready to perfect technique and acquire physical qualities that are specific to their sport or required fitness.

Adults	above 17/18, 18/19

With the onset of puberty there are some profound changes in development, which can throw up some unusual and challenging situations regarding physical capacities in groups of children of a similar age. You can see the early or accelerated children who can excel and the late developers who could seem several years behind them in the same class. The situation will combine the skills of the instructor to control the class levels and of the kids themselves to gauge the level of intensities required of them.

During endurance training in children and adolescents it is vital to understand that the anaerobic capacity hasn't fully developed, and the choice of intensities and the dosage of efforts and time spent in zones must be administered carefully according to the biological development of the individuals. Care must also be taken not to overtrain the children so that they use up the carbohydrate reserves needed for the organs dependent on glucose, such as the brain.

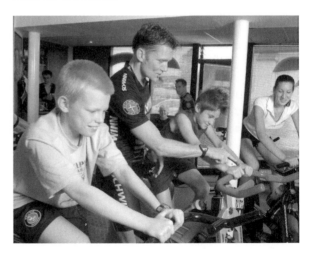

The inactive or normal child's body will adapt to a usual lifestyle level of activity; however the rate of adaptation is slower than that of the active child. After only one week of exercise there are functional changes in muscles; changes in bone, cartilage, tendons and ligaments appear after several weeks. Therefore structured training progression needs to be designed to allow for safe adaptations. In the first few weeks the level of frequency, intensity, time and type (FITT) should be kept at a consistent and safe amount for all the different physical abilities.

Height guidelines:
Unfortunately many studio-cycling bikes have been built for adults or taller children, and it is important to ensure a correct and safe fit for all riders. Anyone below 4ft 8in could have a problem, so although there is no specific age limit, the size of rider will limit inclusion in junior classes.

Disclaimers:
It is just as important for a child and guardian/parent to sign a disclaimer as with normal fitness club members. Make sure it covers all the relevant points and that correct signatures and dates are obtained (see Fig. 2.8).

The rules

Provide a height restrictor for the children to stand next to before the class to satisfy the instructor that they are tall enough. If they are borderline, then the usual simple 3-point saddle-height check is necessary (see Chapter 2, under 'Bike set-up', the 'Quick Fit').

At puberty, with the hormonal changes, muscle mass is considerably increased, with a marked difference between the sexes. Male muscle mass increases to approximately 41.8% whereas female muscle mass increases to 35.8% of total body mass.

Children show different characteristics from adults in their relationship to anaerobic and aerobic capacities. Puberty marks the onset of increased anaerobic capacity but lactic acid production is limited and will not fully develop until between 20 and 30 years old. This underdeveloped anaerobic capacity is compensated by a larger aerobic or oxygen metabolism. This in turn allows muscle cells to

use fatty acids more rapidly than in adults and the glucose reserves are stored well (Berg 1980, p. 490).

Metabolism

The metabolic rates in children will be an extremely important consideration for instructors and coaches and the education of parents and teachers who oversee and advocate exercise for children. With growth spurts and cellular construction these transformations can elevate the metabolic base 20–30% higher than in normal adults, which calls for increased vitamins, minerals and nourishment. The protein intake for a growing child would be increased to as much as 2.5 kg of protein per kg of body weight – as much or more than for an athlete in training for strength events. The metabolic process or catabolism that contributes to energy output during training could cause metabolic construction (anabolism) to predominate and thereby impede growth. Studio-cycling efforts could result in decreased capacity for intensity, and therefore it would be important to allow for adequate recovery not only during classes but between exercises. These recovery periods would help prevent the increased risk of injury. Children lack the strength and endurance of adults.

Children produce less sweat than adults and sweat occurs at a higher core temperature. They will need more time to acclimatise in hot conditions and their core temperature will increase more rapidly than that of an adult because of a poorer ability to perspire, which will reduce performance capacity.

Heart rate

A child's maximum heart rate is often measured at over 200 bpm, higher in females. This is because the cardiovascular system is not fully developed until a later age; however, the Heart Zone rule is the same as in adulthood – maximum heart rate is genetically determined. There are great benefits from training in the different zones. Cardiac muscle fibres in children grow in size with training. The amount of fibres stays the same during growth but they will increase in length and width. The heart rate decreases as the fibres lengthen. The internal heart cavity increases in volume as a result of training and regular growth which in turn increases stroke volume. Cardiac workload becomes more effective and economic. Children's and adolescents's cardiac systems will react similarly to those of adults.

There is no danger to children who do endurance training. Research by Mausberger (1973, p. 52) showed cardiac volumes improved from 12 ml/kg in normal children to 14.9–18.1 ml/kg body weight of children who trained for endurance. This corresponded to heart size statistics of adults. Oxygen consumption also improved from 40–48 ml/min/kg to 60 ml/min/kg. The development of performance capacity in endurance has a strict correlation with cardiac volume and maximum oxygen consumption (from Hollman–Bouchard 1970, p. 160). This shows that endurance training will have the biggest benefits in children, demonstrating that studio cycling can be of great importance as it can be done in a controlled environment and measured and monitored. It will result in a higher performance capacity, guaranteeing protection and maintenance of overall health, a strong immune system and a higher resistance to infection.

Rate of perceived exertion

Studies of the rate of perceived exertion (RPE) in relation to heart rates in children have shown that they are less likely to have a subjective perception of this relationship than adults, even though some adults cannot recognise it without practice. But for an instructor who is a good communicator it can be fun, informative and very useful for control of the class and individual children.

For simplicity the RPE scale 1–10 will link to heart rate percentages 1–100 in Table 11.2.

A healthy heart is a heart that responds

Table. 11.2	RPE in relation to heart rates in children	
Scale 1-10		% of max heart rate
1	asleep	10
2	waking up and getting out of bed	20
3	walking around	30
4	brisk walking	40
5	fast walking	50
6	light jogging	60
7	running, in control	70
8	running fast, hard but sustainable	80
8.5	very hard but sustainable	85
9	very, very hard; fatiguing after seconds	90
10	maximum, too hard!!!	100

quickly to exercise and children normally have the ability to move through the zones faster than adults and make quicker adaptations to stress. The more responsive the heart the fitter it is. We can use this to our advantage and play fun and exciting games with the heart rate responses. You will see below how the games include challenges to move from one zone to another, and there is always a progressive element to each class. At the beginning of each class it is important to explain the programme and its goals. We can create key elements of imagery and visualisation; they can be interwoven within the technical aspects of progression. At the end of each class the teacher can celebrate with the children by implementing a reward structure. For example Heart Zone training points, give-aways or medals.

Note: Most children will not be able to afford a heart rate monitor. Heart monitors have come down in price and an investment of 10–15 entry level heart monitors will be money well spent. They can be placed in station bags designed for the purpose with pouches to carry the watches, belts and straps. This way it makes it easier for the instructor to see if they have all been returned at the end of the class.

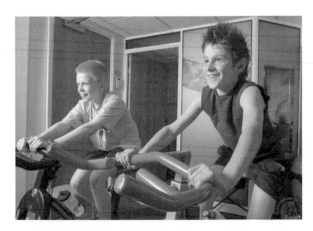

It has been said that children who are below a certain age should not bother to use heart rate monitors as the heart is continually changing up to the ages of approximately 13/14 for girls and 14/15 for boys. However it could equally be said that this tool can become an educator, allowing the children to learn about heart rate responses and use the monitor for interesting and motivating games. As you can see in Chapter 4, Heart Zone Training, the tests can be continually repeated which gives useful up-to-the-minute information that can be correlated and used productively by the instructor/teacher for coaching with use of logbook work.

Children's guidelines (touch, feel, experience!)

Safety

Studio-cycling bikes aren't toys. It is important not only to talk about the fixed wheel and how to slow the legs with the braking mechanism, but also to give the children a practical demonstration on the bike, allowing them to touch and rotate the flywheel (easy) then the pedals (hard). Moving the 17.5 kg weight will be impossible for some kids which will bring awareness of the dangers of stopping pedalling with the legs. They must understand that they have to continue to pedal throughout the class, using the brake and not their legs to slow down. Play the touch game and ask for feedback: 'What do you feel when you do this?'

Towel and water

Hydration in children is even more important than in adults, purely because children are more likely to get excited and forget to drink. In the Rookie class it is important to instil the rules that include: NO WATER OR TOWEL NO SPIN! Try to ensure that every child has a bottle they can fill and that they start to drink before the class. Many children will come to class dehydrated and, just as with adults, their enjoyment will be affected. The rules are: Drink before you ride! Drink while you ride! Drink after you ride! Think Drink Drink Drink!

The towel is to wipe the sweat off both for reasons of hygiene and to stop little hands from slipping off the handlebars.

History of exercise, fitness and health

No child should train when they have an infectious illness such as catarrh, influenza, sore throat, mumps, measles, tonsillitis, or sinusitis. If endurance or speed training is continued with these frequent illnesses there can be serious repercussions such as myocardial or endocardial inflammation. Coordination and movement can be trained and so can strength, in moderation. In tonsillitis and chronic sinusitis, speed and endurance exercises are contra-indicated as they can provoke other bacterial illnesses which are dangerous to the heart. The body will produce antibodies, which will attack the cardiac muscle (Klienman 1980, p. 2520). Illness aside, there will still need to be different levels of class to ensure correct time and durations are observed depending on fitness levels and experience. The child's body is highly trainable during the period of accelerated growth but is also very sensitive to training above its tolerance level. Children must spend a specific time in each phase before they move to the next phase within the same group.

Young bones are more flexible and less resistant to pressure and traction, which would suggest that cycling would be a more beneficial exercise for a child to take up than running, for example. Tendons and ligaments are not strong enough to support heavy demands. All training must follow sensible and slow adaptation periods to stimulate the muscles' growth and strength.

Flexibility training for children

Many children between 8 and 18 years old have bad posture, whether they practise sport or not. During these years if stretching is taught as part of the exercise process then many postural problems would not become apparent later in life. Education is the key to making this vital form of body awareness part of a lifetime of correct stretching. Stretching should vary from dynamic to isometric.

Types of class

Be imaginative with the names of the classes: unusual names. If you simply call the classes Beginner, Intermediate and Advanced you will not inspire the children to attend and could even put them off. Have some fun and make the names interesting and relevent to cycling. Try to promote cycling as a sport and exercise that is 'cool'. The British Cycling Federation (BCF), governing body to the sport of cycling in Britain, actively promotes children's programmes in this way. Around the world more and more is being done to encourage children to take up the sport. Give them role models – the obvious one today would be Lance Armstrong; however, there are plenty of shining examples of prestigious human beings who inspire even the laziest of children.

Here are some examples and ideas for class names and descriptions:

- Level One Class: *Rookies/First timers* (beginner level). This class is for juniors who have never done a studio-cycling class before and will need to be set up on the bike and shown the basic techniques.
- Level Two Class: *Middle of the Pack/Economy Class* (intermediate level). This class is for quick developers who have completed Level One Class and have quickly learnt the new studio-cycling techniques and are raring to

learn more. Add heart rate and focusing techniques.

- Level Three Class: *Front of the Pack/Presidents/Champions* (advanced level). In this class the children will be happy doing the techniques and will understand the importance of progression to see results.

Revolutions per minute

Monitoring the correct leg speeds and resistance is vital for safety. No children or juniors will pedal faster than 100 rpm. Bone and ligament development in children is not completed until after teenage years and to pedal too fast eccentrically (letting the flywheel pull the legs round) or without resistance is fundamentally damaging. The growth of a child must be allowed to continue naturally and each child will grow at a different rate. Therefore we should limit leg speeds, monitor resistance and use heart rate for our guidelines.

> **Training guidelines**:
>
> Use sustained continuous training and short duration intervals; don't use repetitions to anaerobic level.

Junior structure

Table 11.3 is a structure plan for Junior Class One – use it as your template to build all future junior classes around. You can develop three key systems as the individuals develop, adding and subtracting elements (i.e. rules, guidelines, games) as you use your coaching skills to decide what will work best.

It is important to remember when working with children that they are not necessarily 'small adults', certainly in physical terms, and some may be more mentally advanced than others. They need exercise for physical growth but also for psychological development. This is why studio cycling is such a good form of coaching and helping children develop. We all

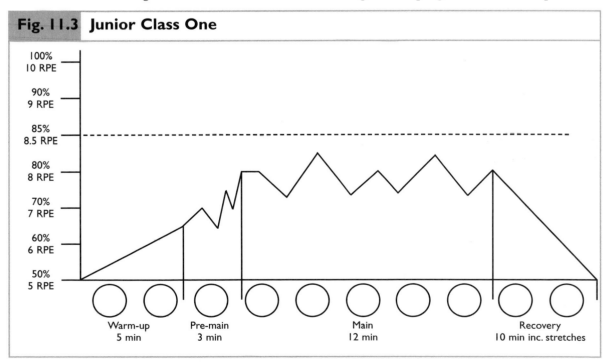

Fig. 11.3 **Junior Class One**

Table. 11.3	'Rookie' class structure sheet	
Things to remember	**Key points**	
Music Sound system Bikes/other equipment Water/towels Rewards Heart monitor station bag	Technique Coaching points Observation Fun games	
Class part	**Elements**	**Notes**
Before class	Safety	Check area for bags, power cables. Ensure towels and water are available. Hand out heart monitors.
	(Game 1, fixed wheel)	Game 1 – feel the flywheel move, look at the pedals, move the pedals, feel the heavy weight. Question – who can feel the heavy weight? Why is it so heavy?
	Rule 1	No one is allowed to stop pedalling otherwise they get left behind and lose points.
	Bike set-up	Use quick-fit bike set-up, to be taught from your bike. Give visual and verbal demos and look for obvious set-up problems. Get class to interact during bike set-up, invite plenty of feedback but stay in control.
	(Option – complete the 1-minute heart zone test)	Use chairs to get the class to sit down and stand up and record heart rate, then use the heart zone guide to rate fitness and find the predicted max heart rate and correct zones column.
Warm-up RPE 5–7 HZ 1–2	Music rhythm	First track playing, used to highlight warm-up. Children should be relaxed and comfortable and look for bike set-up problems.
	Rule 2	Everyone must start with a full water bottle; at the end of the class it must be empty otherwise they lose points.
	(Game 2, give points) Guideline 1	Everyone starts the class with 10 points (good time to go through the RPE scale – keep it simple). The class pedalling speeds are 70–100 rpm on flat roads / 50–80 on hills.
	(Game 3, mimic)	Game 3 is to mimic the instructor and his or her leg speed.

	Hand positions	Explain hand positions on bike and their uses. To be used for variety, posture and introduction of visualisation. Give varied and interesting descriptions to go with each position.
	(Game 4, memory)	Ask the children at the end of the hand positions explanation what they are for – award points.
	Start visualisation (Game 5, where are you?)	Ask group to close eyes if they want to and imagine a place that is familiar to them in a nice environment. Use positive suggestions, with a goal at the end. Set the scene, making it as vivid as you can. Be humorous and include something strange or out of the ordinary – let the class try and hold the image. Ask them what they saw and where they were.
	Basic sitting + teaching points	Participants should sit towards back of saddle, lengthen spine, relax elbows and shoulders, have head in a neutral position, knees over toes and a loose grip on handlebars. Resistance should be added gradually at rate chosen by them. Hands in position 1 or 2.
	Biomechanics – Game 6	Leg action games – ask the children to add resistance and pedal slowly. Run through the biomechanics, breaking down the pedal stroke. At each part of the stroke the children can put their hands on the working muscle to help them understand the part it plays.
	Basic standing	Group to be adding sufficient resistance that it is hard to pedal sitting down; hands in wide position, in one smooth movement stand out of saddle, hips over middle of bike, saddle tapping bottom; loosen grip, transfer weight through pedals, nose crossing centre line. Only to be taught if group is ready. Emphasise that more rather than less resistance is easier to stand. The more skills you learn the more fun the class!
	Mobilisation (upper body)	Upper body movement exercises designed to mobilise upper body ready for main sets. Not stretching. This will loosen and relax tight and stressed areas such as the neck and shoulders.
Pre-main RPE 6.5-8 HZ mid point zone 2 to ceiling zone 3	Other challenges	Designed to elevate heart rate gradually by adding resistance and prepare the body for following challenges in the main set. Examples include seated or standing climbs, but all designed to suit the ability of the group. Look for tension and other problems within the group, highlighting, relaxing and specific coaching points for each challenge.

149

		Music to be more motivating to highlight different part of class. Use fun music choices.
	Game 7	Be varied with the descriptions. Game 7: Focus on muscle groups, changing intensity, leg speed and resistance to work through the zones.
	Peddling techniques biomechanics	Explained to enhance muscle balance, pedalling efficiency and injury prevention. Coached by breaking down the terms 'push forwards and down, pull back and up' using relative terms such as 'scraping dirt off the foot' etc.
Main RPE 7–8.5 HZ floor of zone 3 to mid-point of zone 4	Other challenges (RPE)	Main part of class still designed to suit the ability of group and is high energy, fun and motivating. Pedalling speeds must follow the guidelines for the terrain with an element of letting the beginner juniors ride at their own pace. Challenges to include seated climbs, standing climbs and downhills, aiming to keep effort levels at a peak. For downhills ensure group bend from the hips, change hand position to narrow grip and go as low as they feel comfortable with reduced resistance, watching for excess speed. Using RPE scale and heart rates to gauge intensities. Observation for technique and how group are coping is essential. Music to change once again to highlight different part of class and challenges. Use the five senses and keep the sixth sense to decide if they are coping.
	Game 8	Give the juniors a challenge that motivates them: for instance choose music that is popular and maybe different with a theme, such as rescuing a princess from a castle, or fighting secret agents, with chases etc.
Recovery RPE 7–5	Upper body stretch (on bike)	After main set music changes to highlight recovery and upper body light stretches done on bike to include biceps, triceps, upper back, chest, neck.
HZ floor of zone 3 to floor of zone 1	Lower body stretch (off bike)	Get group off bikes, lower body stretches to include hip flexors, gluteus, hamstrings, quads, upper and lower calf. Stretches done off bike to be more specific with technique and highlight a separate part of the class, which is very important. Time to run through the class profile, count up the points and celebrate with the winners!
	Clean bikes	Juniors to wipe their own bikes down.
Finish	Logbook	Children to fill in their class logbook, learning how to read work-outs and start to plan their own classes.

know that they have a relatively short attention span, so what better way than to place them on stationary bikes next to their friends in a confined space. This form of exercise is safe and effective. They can ride at their own level. However, unlike adults, they need more monitoring as they can become too competitive. A child adapts to training very differently throughout the various stages of adolescence, the metabolic rate has a higher base rate than that of an adult, and therefore there is a need to increase nourishment and to follow a closely monitored diet. Perhaps the key to coaching children is to capture their attention, whether by means of a competition ride where they win prizes at the end, or a class where they have the chance to ride as a hero of their choice. Work *with* the children, do not allow them to overtrain, and you will be helping to build our athletes of the future.

Seniors

Ageing is part of life. We are unable to change how we look, it is a natural process that everyone

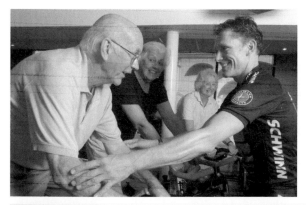

Fig. 11.2 Age groups in terms of percentage of world population

must go through. However, we *can* choose our quality of life by looking after ourselves in the best way we know how. Just like the juniors, we can improve our motor skills, coordination, endurance and strength. The population of over 50s, 55s, 60s and 65s is growing. The trends are staggering and the number of elderly is increasing each year, causing social structures to

Table. 11.4	Percentage of dependent populations of the world			
Age Groups	1975	2000	2025
Younger than 15 years	37	30	24
Older than 65 years	6	7	10

change. The fitness industry is somewhat behind, but catching up fast. It has realised that there is a whole new market of potential older members to aim for and attract into their clubs. So large is this market that the whole approach to health clubs is changing. Even now, 40% of health clubs' members are over 60, so more and more studio-cycling classes must cater for this vital and expanding group of highly motivated individuals who should have more than just a small voice.

A health club must appeal to this special population group by designing an atmosphere that is attractive to train in (no big weight rooms full of body builders!) with creative classes aimed at the right level and taught by instructors who understand the physical, psychological and social requirements of this very important market.

Studio cycling is now putting together senior classes aimed at providing almost the same benefits as younger classes but with a totally different approach, with goals modified appropriately.

Studies on life expectancy show that more and more people are reaching old age. Medicines, health care, diets, exercise are all contributing to current figures of around 580 million people in the year 2000 and estimates of 1000 million by 2020. Projections for the increased numbers and proportions of older persons are impressive. Between the years 2000 and 2050 the worldwide proportion of persons over 65 years of age is expected to more than double from the current 6.9% to 16.4%. The proportion of oldest-old (those aged 80 years and older) will increase during this period from 1.9 to 4.2%. The population of centenarians in 2050 will be 16 times larger than that in 1998 (2.2 million compared to 135,000) with the male-to-female ratio of centenarians falling to approximately 1:4.

In Italy, which has the largest over-60s population in the world at around 24%, it is expected that by 2050 nearly 41% will be over 60 years old. In the United States the over-60s currently comprise 16% of the population; by 2050 it will be 28%.

A 1999 survey of cycling in the UK found that 2.3 million bikes had been sold, whereas Germany had sold 4.71 million. There are approximately 18,000 competitive cyclists in the UK. The BCF (British Cycling Federation and CTC (Cycle Touring Club) expect these figures to rise, not just because people are living longer but also because governmental policy is to attract more and more people, including seniors, to ride bikes. Studio cycling has an important role to play in this as it can develop core fitness and confidence in all kinds of people to progress to riding outdoors. The NSCR (National Studio Cycling Register), which trains fitness instructors in Britain and Europe, aims, through its instructors, to attract thousands of fit and getting fitter indoor riders who will eventually aspire to buy bikes and ride outdoors. This sits well with government and Sustrans (www.sustrans.co.uk) who are providing a network of cycle paths around Britain for cyclists to enjoy their pastime in a safe and traffic-free environment.

The fitness industry membership in terms of national population is still relatively small, at around 5%. This figure is growing steadily but not fast enough for the large businesses who own and run the corporate chains that can have 50 to more than 100 clubs nationwide. Probably the best and most lucrative market to attract will be the over-60s as they have the time and money to exercise. Social trends are for healthy lifestyles and so they will be more receptive to the clubs that are specifically marketing to them.

There exists a 'win-win' situation, so it is up to organisations and instructors to provide the ideal facilities that seniors want.

In looking at goals for the elderly, we also

Table. 11.5	Age classifications
Term	**Age**
Juniors, adolescents	15–30
Age of maturity	31–45
Middle age	46–60
Elder people	61–75
Older people	76–90
Oldest people	90 +

consider other factors such as social and psychological. The older people get the more society belittles them, labelling them, for instance, as 'over the hill'. Everyone should be allowed to grow old gracefully, so let's break this mould and see how to motivate the elderly. Some may be alone if a partner has died; they could be lonely or depressed. By improving their fitness and health, their well-being improves, which in turn brings social benefits such as contact with other like-minded people.

Other benefits which can improve quality of life in seniors concern correlations between physical activity and better mental health, less depression, reduced anxiety, higher tolerance of stress and improved self-esteem. A study done in 1993 by O'Conner *et al.* showed this was because exercise reduced depression by raising confidence. In fact, physical exercise can be prescribed for anxiety, muscle tension and stress, but it is actually aerobic exercise that combats anxiety.

Cognitive changes associated with age are increased short-term memory losses although long-term memory is often good. Learning is not a problem; the elderly can be taught new physical skills and will retain this information at a higher level than normal if exercising.

Experience has shown that this learning process can be implemented to great effect in studio-cycling classes if the information is taught when the individuals are working within 55–65% of their maximum heart rate, when they are feeling good, warming up, in control and confident.

Different categories of seniors:
- Sedentary (inactive) Care at the level they start, but will follow the professional guidance due to inexperience.
- Sedentary (ex training) Risk category because they remember how they used to train, can be influenced by younger people who train.
- Trained (currently training) Assess their training level because they have always trained, little risk.
- Athletes (still competing) Compete regularly (more than average) as master athletes.

or
- Fat and fit
- Fat and unfit
- Thin and fit
- Thin and unfit.

Physical activity, health and ageing go hand in hand. Not that the more somebody trains the less they age or the healthier they are, but the better quality of life they may experience. With a balanced regime of exercise it is quite likely that a person will continue to be more active as they get older. However, the older you get the more chance you have of chronic illness that will prevent exercise – so it can be a vicious circle. The goal is to stay active, as it will have a positive effect on functional ability and health.

Studies with persons over sixty show:
- A reduction in physical activity will start a diminution of the thin muscular mass.
- A reduction of the area of the muscular fibre.
- A reduction in the total number of fibres.
- Diminution of the basal metabolism and increase of fat mass.
- Definitive loss of muscle mass after 30 years (average 1% per year).
- Strength training is still beneficial even up to the age of 90, strength gains of as much as 100% are possible.
- Loss of muscle strength is connected to hormone level, especially testosterone.
- Bone formation is continual at a faster pace than the reduction of bone until peak bone mass is reached at the approximate age of 30. After that, bone reduction begins to exceed bone formation.
- With ageing there are signs of wear in most joints, especially in the knees, hips and ankles: this is called arthrosis. It is often defined as arthritis.
- Osteoporosis is normally another sign of old age where the bones become more fragile and more likely to break. Typically this occurs in the spine, hips and wrists.
- In the US 10 million individuals have osteoporosis.
- US national expenditure for osteoporosis-related treatment is $14 billion each year.
- In Germany this figure is approximately 7 million people resulting in costs of 1 billion Euro.
- Studies have shown that osteoporosis can be stopped, even in old age.

Cardiovascular changes with ageing

Ageing and its associated reduction in activity could also be the reason for cardiovascular deconditioning. This can be modified positively by increasing the level of activity. Sedentary lifestyle affects the ability to consume oxygen in the same proportions as muscular loss. A 60–70-year-old can improve the V02 max by 30% with exercise as well as hormonal and immune system functions.

The primary function of the respiratory system (breathing is gas exchange where oxygen is inhaled and carbon dioxide is exhaled) is to supply the blood with oxygen so that the blood can deliver it to all parts of the body. The average adult's lungs contain 600 million spongy, air-filled sacs that are surrounded by capillaries.

Changes with age:
- Decreased pulmonary ventilation capacity and maximum pulmonary ventilation
- Decreased gaseous exchange at the alveolus pulmonary level
- Decreased breathing acts, amplitude 35%

Cardiovascular diseases are the biggest cause of death worldwide in older men and women. Coronary heart disease and strokes are major causes of death and disability in ageing men and women: over 80% of cardiovascular disease deaths occur in people over 65.

In the US more than 960,000 people die of cardiovascular disease each year, accounting for 40% of all deaths. About 58 million Americans live with some form of cardiovascular disease. Heart disease is the leading cause of premature, permanent disability among working adults. Strokes alone account for disability among more than one million people nationwide. Congestive heart failure is the single most frequent cause of hospitalisation for people aged 65 and older. Cardiovascular disease costs America $274 billion each year, surely a good reason to start a studio-cycling training programme. It is one of the best forms of cardiovascular training within the fitness industry.

Arteriosclerotic cardiovascular diseases include coronary heart disease (CHD); stroke; peripheral arterial disease (PAD). The heart needs a constant supply of oxygen and nutrients from the blood via the coronary arteries. When these arteries become narrowed or clogged and can't supply enough blood to the heart, the result is cardiovascular disease. If not enough blood reaches the heart the heart responds with pain, known as angina.

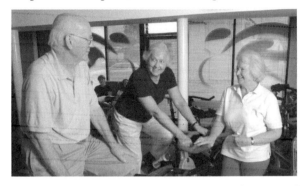

By the age of 70 the incidence of cardiovascular disease is 15% in men and 9% in women. This increases to 20% by the age of 80 in both men and women. At 90 or older 70% of people have occlusion of one or more coronary vessel. Age has been shown to be an independent risk factor for cardiovascular disease.

A stroke is damage to a part of the brain caused by interruption to its blood supply or leakage of blood outside the vessel walls. Sensation, movement or function controlled by the damaged area is impaired. Strokes are fatal in about one-third of cases and are the leading cause of death in developed countries.

The severity of peripheral arterial disease depends on time of detection and pre-existing health factors, such as smoking, high cholesterol, heart disease or diabetes. Later-stage symptoms can be poor leg circulation causing pain in toes and feet during inactivity, especially at night. This condition needs immediate attention as it could result in amputation if not treated. Part of the treatment process will be exercise and rehabilitation in the form of studio-cycling classes. It will be very important that the instructor taking the class knows what kind of cardiovascular disease or operations the members have had.

After operations, including coronary artery bypass graft, a balloon angioplasty or a coronary artery stent, the patient may feel cured but will still have arteriosclerosis and high blood pressure with raised intensity; with the lightest of cycling their blood pressure will be raised further so it is equally important that special care be taken with these clients. (A stent is often used to support tissues while healing takes place; it is a small, self expanding, stainless steel mesh tube that is placed within a coronary artery to keep the vessel open.)

Constitutional risk factors for getting arteriosclerosis are:
- Age
- Gender
- Race
- Heredity

External risk factors include:
- Smoking (3 times the risk of non-smokers)
- Being overweight (android adiposities – metabolic syndrome)
- Physical inactivity
- Poor diet
- Stress

Internal risk factors:
- Hypertension (high systolic blood pressure) High blood pressure risk factors increase from lowest to highest values for either systolic or diastolic with blood pressure of 130/35 said to be normal and at 140/90 is called arterial hypertension. Elevated blood pressure is associated with external risk factors such as dietary intake, obesity, elevated blood lipids, smoking, diabetes mellitus (type 2) and physical inactivity.

- High blood glucose levels (causes diabetes mellitus)
- High cholesterol levels
- High uric acid levels (causes gout)

High blood pressure is dangerous because it makes the heart work too hard and, without testing, it can be present without a person's knowledge. In Germany it is estimated that 5–8 million people have high blood pressure. In America about 50 million, or 1 in 4 have high blood pressure. By the age of 60 about 60% of Americans have high blood pressure. It is possible to lower high blood pressure by exercising because high blood pressure is often associated with being overweight. An example would be to lower blood pressure 3 mm hg systolic and 2 mm Hg diastolic for every kilo lost. Therefore a person with a blood pressure 170/110, who reduces their weight by 10 kilograms results in a reduction of blood pressure of 140/90 which would be normal to high.

Another way to lower blood pressure is to take medication, although this isn't going to replace positive lifestyle changes. Diuretics flush water and sodium from the body. This reduces the amount of fluid in the blood. Since sodium is flushed out of the blood vessel walls, vessels open wider and the pressure goes down. Beta-blockers reduce nerve impulses to the heart and blood vessels, urging the heart to beat less often and with less force. As the workload decreases, blood pressure drops, especially during physical activity. This means the heart rate may only reach 130–140 beats per minute even with higher intensities. Information about medication is crucial for the instructor and coach of the class.

Diabetes

Almost 16 million people in America have diabetes mellitus. Diabetes is a disorder of the metabolism, the way the body uses digested food for growth and energy. Food is normally broken down into glucose in the form of sugar in the blood. After digestion, glucose passes into the bloodstream where it is used by cells for growth and energy; for this process there must be insulin present, which is produced by the pancreas. People with diabetes either do not produce enough insulin or the cells do not respond properly to the insulin that is produced. Glucose builds up in the blood and overflows in the urine, and the body loses its main source of energy.

There are two types of diabetes: Type 1 is an autoimmune disease that results when the system for fighting infection turns against a part of its own body. In diabetes the immune system attacks and destroys the insulin-producing beta cells in the pancreas so that production is seriously affected. Anyone with this type of diabetes will probably have to take insulin daily for the rest of their lives.

Type 2 is the most common form of diabetes affecting about 90–95% of sufferers. It may develop in adults over 40 but is most prevalent in adults over 55. Of people with this type, 80% are overweight. Symptoms often include obesity, elevated blood pressure, high levels of blood lipids. This is becoming more and more common in children and young people as they are statistically becoming less active and more overweight. In type 2 diabetes it would appear that the body produces enough insulin but doesn't utilise it properly. Diabetes can lead to blindness, heart and blood vessel disease, strokes, kidney failure, nerve damage and amputations. Instructors should look for signs of both hypoglycaemia (blood sugar deficiency) and hyperglycaemia (too much blood sugar). If suspected medical assistance should be obtained and in the case of a deficiency, the member should be given fast carbohydrates in the form of sugar or juice.

High cholesterol levels can be lowered.

Blood lipids (fat in blood) are composed of cholesterol, tryglyceride, phospholipid and free fatty acid. Hyperlipidemia is the presence of excess fat in the blood and can imply high cholesterol and trygliceride in the plasma and is linked to arteriosclerosis. There are five different sizes of lipoproteins and of the five the two most important and talked about are the HDL (high-density lipoproteins) and LDL (low-density lipoproteins); the balance of these lipoproteins has to be right if cholesterol is to be excreted from the body. LDLs are overloaded with cholesterol and HDLs have a third to half as much. However, they seem to have the ability to pick up cholesterol left behind by the LDLs. Excess cholesterol causes irritation and the body responds with inflammation, damage and scarring. This can result in strokes and heart attacks, as blood cannot flow unimpeded through the arteries. The high levels of cholesterol are not the main problem but rather the proportion between the two, HDL and LDL. This can be improved by doing low end endurance exercise, 65–75% of max, as well as making positive lifestyle changes, cutting out smoking, excess alcohol, stress and inactivity.

Respiratory tract diseases

1 Bronchial asthma
2 Chronic obstructive pulmonary disease
3 Lung emphysema

Some 100–150 million people in the world suffer from **bronchial asthma**, and this figure is rising dramatically every year. The symptoms are varying degrees of breathlessness and wheezing caused by inflammation of the airway passages in the lungs. The sensitivity of the nerve endings in the airways is affected so they become easily irritated. The lining of the bronchial passages swells causing the airways to narrow and reducing the flow of air in and out of the lungs.

Chronic obstructive pulmonary disease is air-flow obstruction associated with **emphysema** and chronic bronchitis: symptoms include chronic coughs, chest tightness, shortness of breath, increased mucus production and frequent clearing of the throat.

All these diseases must be considered when running classes for seniors as it is possible dramatically to improve the individual's health and fitness with classes that target these groups with the correct duration and intensities. Classes must be designed according to the kind of seniors in the class. Changes can be made to the duration of the class, and there can be choices of techniques that will bring various advantages to the different types of seniors within the class.

Biomechanics

With seniors as with all other studio-cycling classes, pay particular attention to correct pedalling techniques. The class must learn how to pedal correctly, and understand the use of the muscle groups, so that they are comfortable and know what they are doing and why they are doing it. The best time to teach biomechanics will be at the end of the warm-up and at the start of the recovery.

The programmes

Long warm-ups and recoveries are important (studies have shown that seniors may need as long as 30 minutes to warm up); the usual 5–10 minutes is just not sufficient.

Programme 1 – Seniors One

(Sedentary – inactive or ex training).
Guidelines: Classes should start at 25–30 minutes' duration with the programme goal to progress to 40–45 minutes over 8–12 weeks. Control must be kept with the ex-training

seniors to make sure they don't work too hard. After 12 weeks of positive feedback and consistent training they can move on to Programme 2 – Seniors Two (see below).

Use a shortened version of low end endurance classes 1–4 including recovery class and limit techniques to seated flat. This is so that blood pressure is not raised by isometric stress caused when doing seated climbing or standing flat.

Use heart rate monitoring if possible, heart rate guidelines are 50–75%. Use Heart Zone tests to ensure correct max heart rate anchor points. If the class members don't have a heart rate monitor they must use the RPE scale as shown.

Keep individuals within the aerobic energy system.

Use longer, slower stretching at the end of the class to lengthen it to the full 45 minutes. This will improve mobility and flexibility and aid recovery.

Programme 2 – Seniors Two

(Trained and are currently training).
Guidelines: These classes should start at 35–40 minutes' duration with the programme goal to progress to 40–45 minutes over 6–8 weeks. Control must be kept with the ex-training seniors who have moved from Programme 1, to make sure they don't work too hard too soon. After 6–8 weeks of positive feedback and consistent training they can move on to Programme 3 – Seniors Three (see below).

Use a version of low end endurance classes 1–4 including recovery class and limit techniques to seated flat and high end endurance with limitations on technique to seated flat, standing flat, and seated and standing climbs only.

Ensure the use of heart rate monitoring. Heart rate guidelines are 50–80%. Use Heart Zone sub-max cycling tests to ensure correct

max heart rate anchor points to find the five zones. If the class members don't have a heart rate monitor they must use the RPE scale as shown and introduce manual testing during the class.

Keep individuals within the aerobic energy system below 80%, with flexibility routines still observed after the class, but a little more time is spent on the bike.

Programme 3 – Seniors Three

(Athletes still competing regularly).
Guidelines: These classes should start at 45 minutes' duration with the programme goal to progress intensities and durations over 8 weeks. Control must be kept with the training seniors who have moved up to this level to make sure they don't work too hard.

Use low end endurance classes 1–4 including recovery class plus high end endurance classes 1–4, competition classes 1–4 and hill classes 1–4. This is so that blood pressure is not raised by isometric stress caused when doing seated climbing or standing flat; you can include all the techniques except sprints. The benefits, now that the class members have built a base of training, will be to add techniques such as combination flats and hills which will help with coordination, a very important exercise for seniors along with speed of reaction that may prevent trips and falls.

Use heart rate monitoring if possible, heart rate guidelines are 50–85%. Use Heart Zone classes with built-in tests such as the threshold class to ensure correct max heart rate as their anchor point. If the class members don't have a heart rate monitor they must use the RPE scale as shown or manual pulse checks.

Keep individuals within the aerobic energy system.

Use usual stretching routines at the end of the class, continuing to improve mobility and flexibility and aid recovery.

Class music for seniors

Within each programme, tracks must be chosen, considering not just rhythms or bpm, but the type of music. Do not rely on the usual modern music such as trance and pop, but look for old favourites. A little consideration of the seniors' taste in music will make a great deal of difference to their enjoyment. If you have trouble finding suitable rhythms ask the class members. They would probably be only too happy to bring some in for you or give plenty of recommendations. Some ideas might be: ambient and world music; classical for warm-up and recovery, blues, jazz, etc; Beatles' records all have great beats; Elvis, Al Green – the list is endless. All soundtracks, of course, must that have beats that match the bpm and RPM guidelines. A trip to the local library or music store maybe useful where you can listen and count bpm.

The volume of the music must be controlled as older people prefer lower levels and want to hear exactly what the instructor is saying. Use a head microphone and speak slowly, clearly and audibly.

Marketing for seniors

Class timetables can list useful information for senior classes including structured outlines of the type, level and intensity they can

experience. The best way to market to this group is to be informative, list the benefits and appeal to like-minded individuals who can train together in a non-threatening and non-competitive environment.

Seniors are so often seen as individuals that have lived their lives and should now retire and become sedentary. This chapter has displayed that is certainly not the case. Even inactive elderly people can change their lifestyle in order to become healthy and fit; all we need to do is keep a watchful eye on the various types of elderly. You should assess how long they have been training, whether they compete, whether they suffered from any illness. Many people are ashamed or embarrassed to admit that they have been ill; however, it is vital that you discover all medical history. Just because people are getting old does not mean that they have to enjoy training any less, and studio cycling is an excellent way to allow older people to feel as if they are still young. Some older individuals are capable of joining a class not specific to the elderly, where they have the opportunity to listen to popular music in a younger environment, helping morale and well-being. However, this may not suit all elderly people. We all have to get old at some point in our lives, so why not benefit yourself now by getting fit for the future – it may even help you look and feel younger for longer!

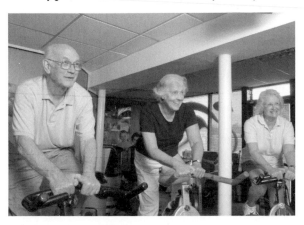

GLOSSARY

Aerodynamic – streamlined position on the bike

Ambient Heart Rate – heart rate throughout the day when the body is awake but inactive

Biomechanics – the correct pedalling technique with muscular recruitment

Cadence – the speed of your legs when they are spinning, measured in rpms

Class profile – diagram showing heart rate techniques and duration of classes

Combination flat/jumping – rising in and out of the saddle in a selected rhythm

Combination hill – rising in and out of the saddle in a selected rhythm with resistance and a selected leg speed

Concentric contraction – the physiological response that shortens the muscles moving the bones towards each other

Criterium – a multilap bike race held on a short course

Delta heart rate – heart rate response to body position change

Double-sided pedals – bike pedals that have a toe clip on one side and use the clipless pedal system on the other

Drive chains – the pedals linked by the chain, the gears and the flywheel

Eccentric contractions – lengthening of the muscle with external forces

Extensive intervals – class heart rate profile between 65 and 85% of maximum heart rate efforts and recoveries in a timed sequence

FITT – Frequency Intensity Time and Type

Fixed gear – the chain drives the flywheel but allows no freewheeling (you must keep pedalling)

Flywheel – specifically designed weighted wheel normally located at the front of a studio cycling bike

Freewheeling – while the flywheel is rotating the pedals can be stopped

Heart Zones™ – universal system working with heart rate monitors and five zones

High-end endurance (HEE) – class heart rate profile between 75 and 85 % of maximum heart rate.

Intensive intervals – Class heart rate profile between 65 and 90% maximum heart rate efforts and recoveries in a timed sequence

Jumping – rising in and out of the saddle in a selected rhythm

Load bearing – an exercise with no impact

Low end endurance (LEE) – class heart rate profile between 65 and 75% of maximum heart rate

LTG – long term goals

Main set – the focal part of the class

MHR – maximum heart rate anchor point to determine Heart Zones

MTG – medium term goals

NSCR – National Studio Cycling Register

Overtraining – extreme fatigue, both physical and mental, caused by training at a level that the body cannot adapt to

Pre-main set – elevating the heart rate with short efforts to the intensities used in the main set

Quickfit – efficient bike set-up for beginners

Recovery – gradual reduction of heart rate and recycling lactic acid

Recovery heart rate – measured heart rate reduction over one or two minutes from peak heart rate

Resting heart rate – measured heart rate when the body is fully rested

Rhythm presses – upper body movements to a musical rhythm

RPE – rate of perceived exertion

Rpm – revolutions of the pedals per minute

Running – standing out of the saddle with an upright body and hand at the back of the handlebars

Seated climb – sitting in the saddle with high resistance or gear

Sitting – seated in the saddle

Spinning – the term used by cyclists to spin the legs fast

Sprinting – increasing the cadence to challenge the body and mind to go up to 110 rpm with resistance

Standing – out of the saddle

Standing climb – out of the saddle with high resistance or gear

Standing flat – out of the saddle with resistance and leg speed for a flat road

STG – short term goals

Threshold – crossover point from aerobic (with oxygen) to anaerobic (without oxygen)

Tour de France – the largest cycling race in the world lasting three weeks in total

V02 – the capacity for oxygen consumption by the body during maximal exertion

Warm-up – building the core temperature and heart rate gradually

REFERENCES

Berg, Keulet Huber 1980, 490

BikeBiz www.bikebiz.com

Bouchard et.a. 1976, Kemper & Vershurr 1987 Klienman 1980, 2520

BreathPlay™, Ian Jackson www.breathplay.com

British Cycling Federation (BCF) www.bcf.uk.com

British Heart Foundation, Morris www.bhf.org.uk

British Schools Cycling Association (BSCA) www.bsca.org.uk

CTC – Cycle Tourist Club ('Bikes not fumes' 1992) www.ctc.org.uk

Ed Burke – Serious Cycling fig 9.1, 161E Burke, Edmund R., Cormichael, Chris, 'Serious Cycling' (Humankinetics, 2002)

Heart Zones® Sally Edwards www.heartzones.com Sally Edwards and Sally Reed. 'The HRMonitor Book' (Velo Press 2000)

Heart Zones UK Limited www.heartzonesuk.com

Mausberger (1973, 52)

National Forum for Coronary Heart Disease foundation www.heartforum.org.uk

National Studio Cycling Register (NSCR) www.internet-spinoffs.com

Joseph O'Connor and John Seymour 'Training with MLP'

Power Bar website 'Nutritional Facts' www.powerbar.com

Robins Anthony – Body language and mentality

Schwinn – much of the research of this book has been done with the help of the Schwinn Schwinn Fitness Academy 'Instructor Manual' 2002 and many of the techniques and names have been taken from their programmes. Other concepts and ideas, however, are those of the author of this book, who takes full responsibility.

Sharp (National Forum for Heart)

Sustrans (www.sustrans.co.uk)

INDEX

ADP (adenosine diphosphate) 12
advanced intervals 110
aerobic metabolism 12
Alps ride 95
ambient heart rate 51
anabolism 143
anaerobic glycolysis *see* lactic acid system
anaerobic metabolism 12–13
anatomy 11–12, 14
arteriosclerosis 155–6
ATP (adenosine triphosphate) 12
ATP-PC system 12–13
Attach ride 98

bikes 14–24
    brakes 15
    buying 5–6
    flywheels 14–15
    maintenance 15–17
    set-up 17–24
biomechanics (pedalling technique) 24–9, 157
body language 41–2, 45
body position 23–4, 29
Boxhill ride 99
breathing 35–6, 111
Breathplay™ 35–6
British Cycling Federation (BCF) 146, 152
British Schools Cycling Association (BSCA) 141
bronchial asthma 157

cadence 26, 45–6, 67 111, 147
calories 1, 54–5, 59
catabolism 143
Chiltern Hills ride 94
cholesterol levels 156–7
chronic obstructive pulmonary disease 157
class profiles 64, 87–93
    criterium class 94–100
    recovery ride 87
    rolling roads of England 87–9
class programmes 13–14
class structure
    45-minute class 69
    class breakdown 60–3
    class environment 64–7
    fitness elements 64–5
    hills 65
    music 67–8
    planning signs and maps 68–9, 80–1

training zones 59–60
type A class 69, 70
    profile 73
    structure sheet 71–2
type B class 69, 70
    profile 76
    structure sheet 73–5
type C class 69, 70, 76
    profile 79
    structure sheet 77–8
coaching 40–7
    and communication 40–3
    and mental training 40
    and motivation 43–7
Col de la Core ride 96
Col de Mente ride 97
competition rides 92–3
communication 40–3, 105
coronary heart disease (CHD) 155
corporate studio cycling 113–15
criterium class 94–100
    hill classes 94–6
    intervals 96–100
    Tour de France 94
criterium ride 93
Cycle Touring Club (CTC) 152

delta (orthostatic) heart rate 52–3
diabetes 156

Edwards, Sally 49, 114
Emotional Heart Zones® 114
emphysema 157
energy and energy systems 4, 12–13
equipment 6–8
exercise
    aerobic 59–60
    anaerobic 60
    eating and 1, 4
    and recovery 3–4
    zones 54
extensive intervals 96–8

feedback 41–3, 67, 103
fitness 1, 8–9, 21, 64–5
FITT (frequency, intensity, time and type) 44, 136, 142
focus programmes 39, 40
focusing, advanced 110–11

goal setting 43–4, 45, 112
Goldberg, Johnny ix
goniometer 23

health benefits x-xi, 87, 90–1
health concerns 36–7
heart disease 139–40, 154, 155
heart rate 50–3, 55–8, 59–60, 143–4
heart rate monitors (HRM) 7–8, 42, 107–8, 123, 145
   use of 48–9
   and weight management 54–5
heart zone training 48–58
   benefits 50
   exercise results 54
   zone characteristics 51
Heart Zone Training® 50–1
Heart Zones® 49, 114–15
high end endurance rides 90–2
hill classes 94–6
history ix-x
home cycling
   Phase One 123–4, 125–6
   Phase Two 124, 127–8
   Phase Three/10 turbo sessions 124, 126, 127–34
hydration 4, 7, 145
hypertension 155–6

illness
   and injury 138
   and juniors' training 146
injuries 11
   and illness 138
   prevention 23–4, 136
   rehabilitation 116, 139
intensive intervals 98–100
intervals 65, 96–100, 110

Jacuzzis 138
juniors 140–51
   cadence 147
   class structure 147–51
   class types 146
   flexibility training 146
   growth 141–3
   guidelines 141–3, 145–6, 147
   heart rate (MHR) 143–4
   hydration 145
   illness 146
   metabolism 143
   RPE 144–5
   stretching 146

lactic acid system (anaerobic glycolysis) 12–13
leg speeds *see* cadence

logbooks 108
London to Birmingham ride 89
London to Brighton ride 89
Lovers Loop ride 91
low end endurance rides 88–9
lower body stretches 63, 82–3, 85–6, 119
Luz-Ardiden ride 98

marketing 106, 113, 159
massage 138
medical history 8
medical questionnaire 8–9
Mendip Hills ride 95
mental training 38–40, 67
metabolism 12–13, 59, 143
MHR (maximum heart rate) 49, 50–1, 143–4
   tests 55–8
Milan-San Remo ride 92
motivation 43–7, 67, 68
Mount Palamar ride 97
Mount Pego ride 99
muscles 10
   and flexibility 81–6
   stretches 82–6
music 67–8, 69, 79, 111, 159

National Studio Cycling Register (NSCR) 152
nutrition 1
   carbohydrates 1–2, 4
   eating and exercise 1, 4
   after exercise 59
   fats 1, 2–3, 4
   hydration 4, 7
   and metabolism 12
   minerals 4
   protein 1, 3
   vitamins 4

off-bike teaching 109
off-bike training 118–22
overtraining 136–8
Oxford to Cheltenham ride 88

pace line intervals 65
Paris-Roubaix ride 91
peripheral arterial disease (PAD) 155
physiology 12–14
PNF (Proprioceptive Neuromuscular Facilitating)
   stretches 82, 121–2
pregnancy 138, 139
professionalism 102–3
programmes
   corporate 115
   focus 39, 40

seniors 158–9
Public Performance Licence (PPL) 69
pyramid training 65
Pyrenees ride 96

Quick Fit set-up 17–22

recovery 3–4, 53, 63–4, 66, 67, 68, 87, 158
overtraining and 137–8
recovery heart rate 53
rehabilitation 116, 139–40
relaxation 39
resistance 111, 119
respiratory tract diseases 157
resting heart rate 51–2
road race high endurance ride 90
rolling roads of England 87–93
competition rides 92–3
high end endurance rides 90–2
low end endurance rides 88–9
rolling roads of England ride 88
RPE (rate of perceived exertion) 42, 49, 55–7, 123,
124
juniors 144–5
running intervals 65

safety issues 8, 101, 102, 145
saunas 138
Schwinn ix, 18
Schwinn Fitness Academy 6
scene-setting 65
scientific set-up 22–3
seniors 151–9
age classifications 153
biomechanics 157
cardiovascular changes 154–6
diabetes 156
marketing 159
music 159
programmes 158–9
respiratory tract diseases 157
set-up 17–24
body position 23–4
Quick Fit 17–22
scientific 22–3
signs and maps 29–34, 68–9, 80–1
special populations 87
cardiac rehabilitation 139–140
injury rehabilitation 139
juniors 140–51
pregnancy 138, 139
seniors 151–9
Spinning® ix
sports teams: training 115–18

spring classics ride 92
sprint intervals 65
Stay in its Tracks ride 100
stress analysis 136, 137
stretching 63–4, 82–6, 121–2, 138, 146
strokes 155
studio cycling
benefits x-xi, xii
concept of xi-xii
corporate 113–15
history ix-x
at home 123–34
innovations 107
launch 106–7
marketing and promotion 106, 113, 159
and other sports 135
training rules 108–12
tried and tested ideas 107
studio-cycling instructions
essential teaching points 101–5
ten goals 100

team building 112, 113, 116
teamwork 45–6
techniques 24–9
advanced 34, 80–1, 107–8, 109–10, 121–2
basic 29–36
biomechanics (pedalling technique) 24–9, 157
body positions 23–4, 29
signs and maps 29–34, 68–9, 80–1
time trials, with visualisation 65
Tour de France 94
ride 93
training
4-week training diary 120–1
advanced 110–12
advanced stretching 121–2
off-bike 118–22
resistance exercises 119
rules 108–12
training zones 59–60
turbo sessions 124, 126, 127–34

upper body movements 34–6, 61, 63, 83–4, 119

visualisation 38–40, 65, 112
at home 123, 124

warm-downs 66
warm-ups 60–1, 66–7, 68, 83, 116, 158
weight management x, 4, 54–5, 59
Winter Hill ride 90